AVOIDING LIFE MALPRACTICE

Avoiding Life Malpractice

A Physician's Primer on Finding, Evaluating, and Negotiating an Employment Contract

Jared Barton, MD, MPH
and
Michael Van Bibber, MD

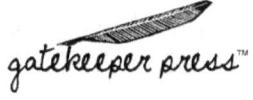

Columbus, Ohio

The views and opinions expressed in this book are solely those of the author and do not reflect the views or opinions of Gatekeeper Press. Gatekeeper Press is not to be held responsible for and expressly disclaims responsibility of the content herein.

Avoiding Life Malpractice: A Physician's Primer on Finding, Evaluating and Negotiating an Employment Contract

Published by Gatekeeper Press
2167 Stringtown Rd, Suite 109
Columbus, OH 43123-2989
www.GatekeeperPress.com

Copyright © 2021 by Jared Barton, MD, MPH and Michael Van Bibber, MD
All rights reserved. Neither this book, nor any parts within it may be sold or reproduced in any form or by any electronic or mechanical means, including information storage and retrieval systems, without permission in writing from the author. The only exception is by a reviewer, who may quote short excerpts in a review.

Library of Congress Control Number: 2021933025

ISBN (paperback): 9781662910814
eISBN: 9781662910821

Contents

Book Organization	7
Why You Need This Book	9
Chapter 1: Finding a Job and Understanding the Players	15
Chapter 2: What Am I Worth?	23
Chapter 3: Different Types of Physician Employment Models	39
Chapter 4: More Than Salary: Other Monetary Considerations	55
Chapter 5: More Than Money: Lifestyle Considerations	65
Chapter 6: Things You MUST and MUST NOT Do.	75
Chapter 7: The Art and Science of Negotiation	91
Epilogue	97

Book Organization

This work is meant to be used as a manual, not a novel. You don't have to read chapters one or two to understand chapter three; rather, you can read each chapter individually based on what information you need. While we hope you read it all, we also understand you are busy medical professionals, and sometimes you just want to know how to treat the illness without wading through a detailed discussion of the base pair mutation that led to the amino acid swap in the critical trans-membrane protein that caused the illness to begin with.

Like a manual, this work is not meant to be an exhaustive treatise on each subject mentioned. We hope to treat each topic thoroughly enough that you will be able to critically evaluate job offers and make better decisions, but contracting and negotiating are fields of study unto themselves. No single work could completely address all aspects of this complex process. However, we have uniquely applicable experience. This book is written *by* busy clinical physicians *for* busy clinical physicians. We've compiled for you exactly what we would have liked to know before we signed our first contracts.

So, with that in mind:

Foreword 1: Dr. Barton's story about WHY YOU NEED THIS BOOK.

Foreword 2: Dr. Van Bibber's story about WHY YOU NEED THIS BOOK.

Chapter 1: Finding a Job and Understanding the Players

The players you'll work with throughout your job search and how to manage each of them.

Chapter 2: What Am I Worth?

How to determine and place a value on your services.

Chapter 3: Employment and Practice Models

Contract issues that arise with different employment and practice models and how to address them.

Chapter 4: More than Salary: Other Monetary Considerations

Other benefits besides a salary to consider when signing a contract.

Chapter 5: More Than Money: Lifestyle Considerations

Reviews lifestyle and other work requirements to consider.

Chapter 6: Things You MUST and MUST NOT Do

How to overcome your nature and bias to get the very best deal you can. A list of MUSTS and MUST NOTS that physicians need to consider before starting the process of negotiation.

Chapter 7: The Art and Science of Negotiation

How to negotiate and what traps to avoid.

Why You Need This Book

Foreword 1: Dr. Barton

There is a great story in the bible about Esau and Jacob. Here's the grand-rounds version of the story:

These twin brothers had very different skill sets. Esau, the older, was a hunter. He was red and hairy. Jacob, the younger, was a little more metropolitan and hung out in tents.

After an arduous hunt, Esau returned fatigued from his efforts. He came into the tent to find his younger brother, Jacob, cooking pottage (most likely lentil stew). Esau was exhausted and begged Jacob for the stew. Jacob used this to his advantage and offered Esau the stew on the condition that Esau sold him his birthright in return.

If you're not aware, the birthright was a very big deal; it was a special reward, or blessing, reserved for the oldest son. Isaac, the father to the twin boys, was himself the son of Abraham and, as the birthright heir, had received all from his wealthy and famous father. Isaac loved his oldest son Esau, and Esau was set to receive vast blessings from his father.

However, Esau was famished and said, "I am about to die; of what use is a birthright to me?" Jacob, realizing the value of the trade, happily agreed to the deal, and Esau sold his birthright for the pottage.

It sounds a bit ridiculous, but let's consider Esau's situation. Esau was starving and deprived. He'd been out hunting and thought he was going to die. So, what did he care about the birthright when he thought he was going to starve? He made a poor decision because of his circumstances.

Now ask yourself: Does residency make you tired? As you're finishing this marathon, are you in the correct state of body and mind to negotiate your employment contract? Do you fully understand the consequences of the contract on your future? Do you even have the time to read AND study the contract? What would you trade for a bowl of soup or a guaranteed salary here and now?

In 2012, Jackson and Coker, a healthcare recruiting firm based in Atlanta, studied physicians in their first place of employment. The study found that more than half of physicians left their first job after five years. And, the vast majority of those who departed quit their job in the first one or two years. You'd think that after the knuckle-dragging effort of residency, doctors would love to be out working in the real world. Yet, the number of physicians who leave their first job is larger than all those who quit or transfer from their residency program.

I left my first job after one year. Believe it or not, it was a great job. I loved it—my colleagues were outstanding, the working environment was good, the facilities were immaculate—the list goes on and on. However, my contract was bad. Despite all these good things, I left.

Your residency and specialty training are of great value. Your education and abilities represent the birthright you've earned. Don't give it away because you are tired and aren't informed about what you're getting yourself into. Don't sell your birthright for a mess of pottage!

Foreword 2: Dr. Van Bibber

I finished residency and headed back home to Utah to start what I was certain would be a long and productive career in urology. A year and a half earlier, I'd flown out to interview for this position. The recruiter for the medical group was affable and pleasant, the need for urologic services was obvious, and the standard contract with which I was presented offered more money than anyone in my family had ever made in a year. I'd asked what I thought were reasonable questions about pay, call, and vacation, and everything seemed copacetic. During the next one and a half years, I had a few calls and notifications. The same group was hiring a few other urologists—but there was plenty of work for all of us, I was told. I arrived in Utah and started in practice, assuming that, finally, after all those years of study and toil, I'd be set.

Three years later, I had sold my home in Utah and was driving away from a failed practice, a miserable lifestyle, and predatory partner practices that had made my stay untenable.

How had it all gone so wrong? Wasn't I supposed to be helping others and satisfied in my work? Wasn't I supposed to be comfortable, respected, and successful? Was there some deficit in my medical training? Some gap in my knowledge base that was holding me back? Was I less talented or less capable than the other urologists in town?

After much consideration, I realized that there was indeed something missing. I had failed to protect myself contractually and had failed to recognize what should have been the obvious shortcomings of the practice environment I was joining. I had not taken enough time to scrutinize the contract and had not enlisted any help in reviewing it before signing. I hadn't asked enough questions about the way the practice was managed and about how call was covered in town. I'd failed to realize that an association of physicians of the same specialty where everyone is paid on production is not a team but a conglomeration of competitors. I hadn't realized that my unique skill set was my most important asset and had naively trained these same competitors to perform complex operations, only to have them divert my potential patients once trained. I hadn't taken the time to evaluate the supplemental benefits, or lack thereof, as part of my employment contract and had failed to consider the tax consequences of those decisions.

For years after this experience, I blamed myself. How could I have been so blind? So naïve?

Over the next few years, I had conversations with many physicians and other health care providers with similar stories. I came to realize that, while I had failed in some ways, much of the problem was systemic.

At that crucial juncture, when I was offered and had accepted that contract, I'd had sixteen years of experience after high school in the study of biology, chemistry, physics, anatomy, physiology, and pathophysiology. I'd spent thousands of hours examining patients, taking histories, creating differential diagnoses, and operating on various pathologies. I'd taken on hundreds of thousands of dollars of student debt to get the position I wanted and had lived most of my adult life on part-time wages, student loans, or the meager salary of a resident. I was married, had five children, and was excited by the prospect of a six-figure salary. I had never taken a course or attended a seminar about contract negotiation, accounting, business creation, practice management, or even basic accounting.

My attendings never once talked about signing their contracts or discussed how much they were paid. I'd never researched salary and reimbursement levels and had only a fleeting exposure to correct coding and billing procedures. I believed that my fellow physicians, much like my medical school classmates and resident group, would be a support system on which I could rely once in practice. I believed that the medical group I was joining would be as interested in my success as I was in theirs. I was a resident with a limited salary and only fifteen days of vacation during which I could travel and interview for any job positions. I also felt immense pressure to sign that first contract and have something solid for my family when residency was completed.

And lastly, like many of you, I was a smart guy. Despite my lack of education in business matters and with some degree of naivety, I felt I could figure this out. I could certainly pick through a simple contract and identify any landmines. And with a knowledge of the cost of attorney review, I never seriously considered getting an attorney or a financial professional to check over the contract before I signed on the dotted line.

So, yes, I had failed to protect myself. But it was not that I was careless—the entirety of my educational and life experiences were of almost no use in this situation.

This work is, therefore, our attempt to help physicians make better business decisions and avoid contracting and negotiation errors that could negatively impact their future. It is our hope to provide physicians fundamental, requisite information and resources they will need to protect themselves from an industry that increasingly preys on their inherent altruistic and trusting qualities.

Some physicians will not want or need this book. Some will not care about salary—their trust funds full and inheritances waiting. Others will worry more about their research grants and titles. Idealists will champion the ideal of "the physician as healer" and bury their heads in the sand when the business of medicine is mentioned as if the very talk of remuneration cheapens their noble profession. But for the pragmatic—for those of you who realize that pay, vacation, call schedules, and benefits are not what medicine is really about but do allow the balance in life that will keep you in the practice of medicine well into the future—this book is for you. We hope it helps prepare you for that first contract negotiation. We hope you can use it to build a knowledge base or team to protect you and yours and allow for more stability, wealth, and success.

Chapter 1: Finding a Job and Understanding the Players

The pathway to get into medical school and residency is pretty well delineated. AMCAS and ACGME have these processes wrapped up tight with a nice little bow on top. You complete the requisite courses, spank the MCAT or USMLEs, spend the requisite time filling out your forms, paying your fees, selecting your target schools and residency programs, buying your suit, traveling from heck to breakfast interviewing, and then wait to see where you are accepted.

The job hunt is a completely different animal. There is no centralized platform for physician jobs. There are no centralized forms. There are no up-front fees. Many places will offer to pay for your travel (a nice change!). However, you'll also find that you'll be interviewing and trying to land this job during the busy period of residency, unlike the relatively laid-back time in college or as a fourth-year medical student.

In this chapter, you'll find information to help narrow your job search, find positions of interest, and make first contact with your potential employers. We'll also introduce the cast of characters with whom you'll be communicating and negotiating your contract.

Limit the Search

This is the part of the job process that is actually easiest for many of our clients. Well before the job hunt starts, many physicians have already discussed with their families where they want to live and what type of practice they would like. If you haven't done so already, sit down and discuss it with anyone that you want involved in the process.

Outline and rank the following factors:

1. Geographical location: Where do you want to live? Where does your spouse or significant other want to live? Where do your children want to live? What activities are most important to you and your family? Will you restrict yourself to only one state or region? Are there any states or regions that are clearly off-limits? Are you considering big cities, medium cities, or small towns? What about rural settings? Do you need access to metropolitan areas? What is the cost of living in the areas you're considering?

2. Family: In many ways, this is a consideration of geographical location, but we feel it deserves extra emphasis. Is proximity to extended family important? How close is close enough? How does your family feel about this?

3. Practice goals: Are you looking for a career in academic medicine? Would you like to avoid research but still be involved in teaching students or residents? Are you looking to practice your specialty and leave the ivory tower behind? Do you want to do massive operations and take care of the sickest patients, or will you be okay with transferring the more complicated cases?

4. Reimbursement: How important is your remuneration? We will delve into this with much more detail in later parts of this book. So, for now, just try and provide an honest evaluation of where the money you'll be making ranks in your list of job priorities. If you want to make a boatload and work as an academic physician in a coastal city, something is going to have to give.

5. Workload: Do you plan to work full-time or part-time? Would you consider locums tenens work?

Finding the Jobs

Once you've narrowed the field a bit, you can start to look for specific positions. Most of our clients have found their position in one of three ways: personal connection, staffing service, or web search.

1. Personal connection: Many of the best jobs will never appear on a job listing or employment website. During medical school and residency, you've assuredly made a myriad of connections in the medical field. This is the time to use them to your advantage! You'll find that a call from an attending to their friend at another facility can uncover positions before they are ever posted online. The retirement-age physician that you rotated with during medical school would likely welcome your call to discuss opportunities in their community and may even be willing to discuss an exit if you're planning to come back home to work. Most hospitals and systems will have an in-house recruiter, and a quick phone call might uncover a need that you can fill. You'll never know what is available until you ask—so ask!

2. Staffing services: There are many companies and individuals that exist solely to help facilities fill open positions. These headhunters put physicians looking for work in touch with facilities, and when the jobs are filled, they take home a hefty fee (typically 10–15% of the first year's annual salary) for the placement. If you'd rather have someone else tapping the keys and looking for positions that fit your expectations, these companies may fit the bill. There are a host of large companies and many smaller regional firms as well. The following list is not meant to be exhaustive. But to get you started, here are a few of the more common services:

A. comphealth.com

B. merritthawkins.com

C. weatherbyhealthcare.com

D. locumtenens.com

3. Websites: In the modern era, job opportunities are never more than a few clicks away. A search of your specialty, state name, and jobs will almost certainly return pages of results. The issue with many of these sites is that they don't actually put you in contact with the facilities or practices looking for physicians but with the headhunter companies listed above. Be aware that entering your information on any of these sites may lead to an onslaught of incoming phone calls,

texts, and emails. A few websites to consider when starting your search are:

A. mdsearch.com

B. practicelink.com

C. hospitalrecruiting.com

D. nejmcareercenter.org

E. indeed.com

F. linkedin.com

If you're planning to head to your hometown, hang up a shingle, and start your own practice, the steps above won't be needed. In this case—where instead of finding a job, you plan to create it—we would still advise careful research into the prospective area and needs, and we would refer you to chapter four for important considerations.

Making First Contact

Once you've identified a potential position, you'll typically start with an email or phone call where you and the potential employer will feel each other out in an attempt to make sure their needs and your qualifications are a match. We go into more detail about the art of negotiating in chapter six, but we feel that a brief mention of tactics is needed here.

The contact person you'll deal with is often a recruiter of some sort. They typically have a script and will want to convey a lot of information to you that may or may not be pertinent. You will hear about their payer mix, strong links with the community, dedication to quality care, the new cancer center they just built, the new MRI coming next month, the specialties they've recruited, and their strong financial footing. They'll also tell you that their community has everything you want and is a short drive away from anything that they don't have. They'll be asking you to share information on your interests in their community and in your field of medicine. They'll want to know about your family and will want you to voice your interest in practicing in their locale for years to come.

Having successfully negotiated medical school admission and the residency match, this process will feel very familiar. We would encourage you to treat these steps just like you did the prior admission processes. Listen attentively to their lists of facts. Ask questions that show you are thoughtful and interested. Express enthusiasm that this position is exactly what you are looking for and that you see yourself as a great fit. Remember, at this point of the process, your primary goal is to generate as much interest in you as possible.

If all goes well with this preliminary contact, you will often make arrangements to share some information. You'll send a CV if you haven't already. They might send a boilerplate contract. There will often be some plans made to get you in contact with a few of the physicians in their system.

From here on out, the heavy lifting begins!

The Players

There are a few players you'll meet in the course of your job hunt. We list them here to help you understand the roles of these individuals and to help you remember that every individual with whom you deal has their own motivation that lies outside of your success and happiness.

1. Recruiting agent: These individuals are often working for national or regional firms. They have lists of jobs and lists of providers, and they get paid to put Tab A into Slot B. Remember that these firms are often reimbursed based on your signing a contract, going for an interview, or starting your job. You'll almost certainly never meet them in person, and if you aren't satisfied in your new position, they'll be happy to fill it with someone else (for the same fee) in a few years.

2. In-house recruiter: In-house recruiters are paid employees of the hospitals, clinics, or health care systems that will be courting you. They are often very pleasant and likable individuals who are good at listening and even better at telling you what you want to hear. They are often the point person for communication because of their friendly and personable demeanor, but they typically have no decision-making role. They have no power at all to give you what you want, and once you've accepted an offer, you'll hardly, if ever, see them again. They get paid to show you a good time and get you to sign on the line.

3. CEO: Whatever the setting, this is the individual tasked with making all the parts work together to accomplish the organizational goals. In many settings, they have near-final say on the contract details. They are often very well compensated, and their reimbursement packages may be based on hitting price or quality metrics. They will spin great tales about community needs and their mission, but, in the end, they are often primarily motivated by the fat salaries they glean from the physicians working the fields. You'll often know you're getting close to finalizing a contract when you meet the CEO and they enter the fray.

4. CFO: Chief financial officer. This is essentially the hospital accountant. They often sign the checks, and there are times when you will negotiate with the CFO. Sometimes, the CEO will negotiate a contract with a physician and then come back saying something like, "I ran this by the CFO, and…" For this reason, it's not a bad idea to meet the CFO and talk about the finances and contracts the hospital executes.

5. CMO: Chief medical officer. This individual is typically an employed physician who works as a liaison between administration and the medical staff. They work for the hospital. Because of this, they are often loyal to their employer. This is an important thing to remember when discussing things with the CMO.

6. Board of directors: The board of directors is composed of individuals who represent the hospital. This group has a moral and fiduciary responsibility to carry out the mission of the organization. Any power possessed by the board of directors is really based on the institution they represent. Some hospitals have a board that essentially directs the hospital or health care system, and they are often tasked with appointing the CEO. It is not an uncommon thing to hear about the board but never meet them.

7. Medical staff (chief of staff): These are physicians and sometimes other medical providers that uphold the policies and procedures of the hospital bylaws. They are a group of individuals who participate in credentialing, granting privileges, discipline, and other aspects of managing the hospital medical staff. They are typically providers who donate their time to help make sure the hospital runs and often work closely with administration.

8. Partners: If going to work in a single or multispecialty group, there may be physicians who created, started, or have "bought in" to the practice. They may have a say in which new physicians enter the practice. Review the points made in chapter ten about the relationship between partners, and never assume any of them are looking out for your interests.

Having read the section above, our editor (who does not work in the medical field) asked, "Is there anyone young physicians CAN trust?" The answer is, unfortunately, an anemic yes. You can trust yourself. Beyond that, trust no one, verify everything, and get it in writing. The individuals you are dealing with have interests of their own, and experience has taught us that most will think nothing of sacrificing a few young, idealistic physicians to reach their goals.

Chapter 2: What Am I Worth?

This seems like a fairly simple question: What are your services as a physician worth? If you immediately had a number pop into your head, ask yourself how you came up with that number. Were you thinking only of salary? Were you thinking of an RVU (Relative Value Unit) conversion factor and estimating a specific workload? What benefits did you consider in that internal calculation?

Most physicians come up with a number based on a vague understanding of what colleagues are paid or based on a number that was provided to them from the facility or practice with which they are negotiating. Some might be aware of composite numbers compiled by services that sell their data to health care institutions. For most, however, their expected compensation is based on a guess.

Do you do anything this way in medicine?

You: "Give that patient 50mg of drug A."

Nurse: "Why 50mg?"

You: "I think a friend of mine who works in a hospital in Florida uses about 50mg."

Doesn't that sound absolutely absurd? The decisions you make when asking for a specific salary, reimbursement rate, benefits package, vacation, or call schedule have life-altering effects on you and your family, and just guessing is life malpractice!

In negotiation, there is a term called "anchoring," which describes the practice of one party in the negotiation providing the first number around which the negotiation proceeds. If the hospital where you are interviewing offers $250,000 per year and a signing bonus of $10,000, they are aware that the negotiation is now anchored. You might ask for more. But, if you don't know exactly what you are worth, you will probably accept their anchor as a reasonable starting place and feel good if you move the negotiation in your favor by 5–10%.

In a negotiation, there can be benefits to setting the anchor and benefits to letting your opponent do it for you. Watch an episode of *American Pickers*, and you'll see master negotiators at work. Sometimes, they offer good money right up front to "break the ice," and sometimes, they stall and let the collectors make the first offer. Imagine watching an episode of that show if one party had no idea what that old Harley in the garage was worth!

In medicine, hospitals and practices understand anchoring even if they don't refer to it as such and will almost always plant a firm anchor in hopes of tethering your expectations. If you don't understand what you are worth, if you haven't explored the limits of reimbursement, you won't stray far from the weighted offer that has now sunk to the negotiation floor. And, unlike the *American Pickers*, if you accept a ridiculously low offer, they aren't going to tell you that you're undervaluing yourself and add a few more bills.

To help you understand your value, we will consider all the different ways physicians add value to health care companies, explore the metrics hospitals and health care organizations use to anchor your expectations, review value data on physician services, and discuss querying local physicians.

Ways Physicians Add Value

Imagine that you get a new job as the janitor at a medical clinic, and you were told that your duties included washing the windows, emptying the trash, dusting the desks and computers, mopping the floors, scrubbing the toilets, and vacuuming the waiting areas. You will also be training a new janitor, but since they are in training, you have to redo anything they manage to clean while under your supervision.

Your pay at this new job will be based solely on the number of windows you have washed. All other duties are deemed critically important, but clinic finances do not allow for you to be reimbursed for time spent scrubbing toilets, etc. You protest this pay structure, but your new boss informs you that all of the janitors working there have agreed to this system, and it works out well.

It sounds ridiculous, but many physicians we work with feel compelled to mop the floors and take out trash for free. If you are on a purely production model and the hospital wants you to take call without reimbursement, that is exactly what you are doing. If that is your choice, so be it. But if you feel, as we do, that it is legitimate, reasonable, and responsible to seek compensation for ALL the value you add to an institution, consider carefully the following list when evaluating and negotiating your contract. And, if you choose to work for free, remember that you are not just negatively impacting yourself but many of the physicians who work alongside you and those who will follow you.

Clinical Work

This is almost certainly the type of work that comes to mind when you think of reimbursement. You see patients, perform procedures, document those activities, and get paid to do so. You might have a base salary with an estimation of a certain amount of clinical activity, or you might be in a system where pay is calculated based on collections or where you are reimbursed a specific amount for everything you do (think RVUs).

The amount you are paid for the things you do (often termed professional fees) is negotiated with insurance companies. There has been a significant decrease in these fees over the years. Many doctors compensate for decreasing professional reimbursement by increasing workload. Hospitals and health care systems also push physicians to do more and more to justify salaries, which are often based mostly on these continually declining fees.

Clinical work can also include pay incentives that are based on volume, quality, citizenship, or patient satisfaction.

Unfortunately, for many doctors we work with, clinical work is the only area of value they ever consider when working out a contract.

Call

Although it is often lumped in with clinical work, call is an entity unto itself. Many physicians will sign offers with facilities or groups where they are paid on a strict production model (you are paid solely for your professional production). The same hospital will then turn around and require a certain number of days covering their emergency room or walk-in clinic. When on call, they will tell you that you can see patients, bill services, and make more money. But what about the 24-hour period on call when you don't get called in? Your family might be at the lake or hiking, but you're sitting at home, not being paid a red cent! And what if your pay is based on collections, and the two patients you see and operate on during your weekend on call are uninsured? What if having you available means the hospital can meet the criteria for a level two trauma center and bill more for radiology and other services but not give you more compensation?

Call coverage is incredibly valuable to hospitals. But time on call, whether you're in the hospital or just waiting for your phone to go off, can be quite taxing. Hospital bylaws may require that you take some call as part of admitting privileges, but, in our experience, the physicians who demand to get paid for call and are willing to consider creative alternatives (work with the competitor across town, downgrade to courtesy staff for a period of time, etc.) will usually end up being compensated for call.

Operative

We are not talking about the physician professional payment here; that is included in the clinical section above. Operative value means that every time you take a patient to the operating room for a procedure, there is a separate operative charge or facility fee that is billed by the institution. These fees are negotiated separately from professional fees and are often quite lucrative for hospitals. In the course of writing this book, we made several attempts to evaluate these reimbursement rates and compare rates of change to rates of change in professional fees, but the information seems to be a well-guarded secret. Make of that what you will, but it seems plausible that hospitals could maintain their bottom line by increasing facility fees, lowering professional fees, paying doctors less, and making out like bandits. In addition, for surgeons and proceduralists, operative cases allow institutions to bill for anesthesia units.

Radiology/Lab/Pathology

When logging in to our EMRs, we are often confronted with a page of orders (many that have been entered by our nurses at our behest) in need of signature. A typical busy day in the clinic might be associated with fifty to one hundred such orders: labs, CTs, MRIs, ultrasounds, X-rays, pathology requests. Almost every single order is a billable event for some organization. Anti-kickback laws and Stark laws make it illegal to be reimbursed directly for each scan or lab ordered or to refer such to a separate business in which one has ownership. If you are going to work for a health care organization or hospital with in-house facilities, it is important to realize how much value you add through the ordering of appropriate tests. If they don't hire you, and those same patients see a doctor in another facility, the health care entity loses not just the fees associated with the patient visit but all the ancillary income from the additional tests and studies noted above.

Administrative

We know you can't wait to finish residency and get out into the real world, where you can sit on the Medical Executive Committee and spend hours listening to data and deciding the fate of other physicians working at the hospital! Or the IT committee, where you can decide whether or not the new communications app is best for your institution. In reality, you almost certainly didn't go into medicine to be an administrator, but time spent in committee meetings will be part of the job. You will be exhorted and manipulated into spending your time to help create and adhere to organizational goals and policies, review data, and a myriad of other tasks required to keep a hospital running. Physician participation on these committees is often mandated through bylaws as well as contracts, and most of the committees cannot run without your expertise and medical knowledge. Remember that none of the hospital administrators sitting on those committees is doing it for free.

Teaching/Education

The local medical school has a program with your new hospital to send all of their third-year students through your clinic for one to two weeks a year. You will have the privilege of participating in this program and paying it forward. You will need to spend time between patients explaining your thinking and sharing what you've learned. When clinic is over, you'll need to stay an extra hour or so finishing the notes you couldn't work on because you were teaching. Every one of those students is paying tuition, and you can bet that your institution is receiving some form of compensation for your work in providing that education.

Legal/Governance

One day, you might enter your office to find an official letter from the department head asking you to review a recent case wherein one of your partners had a complication. You are asked to review the notes, labs, and associated radiographs and provide a written assessment of whether or not the standard of care was met in this instance. As a medical professional, you will frequently be called on to help your organization with matters of legal and professional oversight. Do you think a consulting attorney would perform similar services for free?

Recruiting

There are several ways that your skill set can help with recruiting. First, you know other physicians and may provide contact information to your institution as they seek providers. Second, you will be asked to attend dinners, lunches, and meetings to shake hands and sell the institution to prospective providers. Third, your skill set can be a selling point for a doctor looking to join your organization. (If you are a hospitalist, your work to facilitate admissions might be used as a selling point for a prospective orthopedic surgeon. An interventional radiologist may be seen as essential for a urologist or general surgeon looking to join an organization.) Recruiting firms are paid handsomely for the physicians they bring in, and you should be too.

Program Creation/Facilitation

The hospitals or groups you join may be able to pursue specific certifications and status based on your education and qualifications. For example, a general surgeon, orthopedic surgeon, and neurosurgeon may allow trauma certification at a level that allows for increased billing.

Locums reduction

When you take a position with a facility, you may be decreasing their need to augment current services with locum tenens positions. Staffing with part-time or locum tenens physicians is very expensive. Hospitals or organizations will often have to pay for travel, a hotel, a locums company, and the salary of the covering physician. Your work may fill a very pricey void.

Referrals

If you worked selling widgets, you could refer your widget customers to a friend who makes widget covers, and he could reimburse you for the referrals. In medicine, this is against the law. You cannot be reimbursed for referrals. The federal government has recently filed some high-profile cases alleging inappropriate referral patterns.

Health care organizations are not supposed to direct you to send your referrals within a system either. In reality, they often do, through direct or strong indirect methods, but they are good at covering their demands, and they have teams of lawyers to protect them when found out.

With that being said, your referrals to others in your organization are a major source of income for the institution, and you should know this.

To summarize: You do a lot. Demand payment for everything you do. No one else will demand it for you! A production model that pays you only for clinical work, collections, or RVUs means you are cleaning floors and emptying trash cans for free.

Value/Reimbursement Metrics (MGMA and others)

> Get your facts first, and then you can distort them as much as you please.
> —Mark Twain

"I'm sorry, Doctor Jones. We can only offer you a salary that is within MGMA established guidelines." If you plan to do any medical contract negotiation, this is a sentence you will hear. So, what is MGMA? Why does it limit reimbursement? Is it valid in all areas and circumstances?

In short, there are companies that make their money by helping hospitals (and physicians, supposedly) decide what amount physicians should get paid. The Medical Group Management Association, or MGMA, is one of these companies. In general, they provide an average compensation for a given specialty to a health care facility or physician, which acts as a base around which negotiations proceed.

We will address the many different payment models for physicians in Chapter three, but for now, consider an example of a pure salary position and think of MGMA as the number the hospital will offer in their first salvo. This number can feel quite powerful, as it seems to be widely accepted, but, as we will show you below, it is simply a derived statistical number. And, as our previously quoted Mr. Twain was fond of saying, "There are lies, damned lies, and statistics."

MGMA. This is a national association of administrators that produces a physician compensation survey. The data from this survey can be purchased by physicians and physician employers for guidance with physician salary offerings. MGMA has reported that their report is compiled "representing data from more than 147,000 physicians and non-physician providers in over 5,500 organizations."

MGMA data sets can be queried to provide data on provider compensation, on-call compensation, provider placement or starting salaries, academic compensation, and other factors. They also offer tools for what they term "data-dive" that would allow you to access information by specialty and even to break things down into rural and urban areas.

In practice, data diving is rarely done. Surveys of large swaths of physicians are taken, data is compiled, a mean is kicked out, and you are presented with that number as fact. You then start your negotiations with that mean number as the anchor. You will almost never see the source data, of course. You will be unlikely to dive into the data and try and account for practice type, geographic location, time in practice, etc.

As a physician or practice, you can join MGMA and get access to these reports. In our experience, no individual physician has ever done this as they prepare to negotiate salary, though there are surely some overachievers.

Why?

To be fair, we are not sure. It is likely time and cost-prohibitive for many physicians. Others are likely trusting of the numbers provided.

MGMA is used extensively by hospital administrators and physician recruiters in offering employment salaries. MGMA's website touts their data as a way for hospitals to make sure they are providing fair compensation packages to attract top talent. In reality, we see MGMA and other metrics used far more often as an "authoritative" cap to limit salary and other demands. It's almost always the same "I'm sorry, Doctor Jones" dialogue mentioned above.

In our experience, the salary number offered up is almost always the MGMA average. You'll occasionally see an offer for the 60th percentile of MGMA, but almost never an offer for 75% or higher. We would remind you that these are often NATIONAL averages, and the price paid for services in sunny San Diego or at an academic institution should have no impact on what you can demand at a private hospital in the frozen tundra of the Midwest.

As physicians, we are constantly scrutinizing data. We rely on this skill to make management decisions for our patients. Do you accept the results of trials based only on the abstracts, or do you dive into the data and do your best to confirm the validity of the information you are receiving? Why wouldn't you do the same when evaluating the data that went in to determining your salary? So, if your potential employer provides you with an "MGMA average," find out as much as possible about what inputs they provided to generate that number.

MGMA is not the only service that accumulates and disseminates physician reimbursement data. Here are few others:

Sullivan, Cotter, and Associates: Another firm that distributes surveys to physicians to determine doctor salaries. Results are generated for providers, administrators, and health care staff. These surveys have been around for over twenty-five years and have a very similar setup as MGMA. One has to pay to receive the data from their survey(s). It is not used as extensively as MGMA by hospital physician recruiters.

AMGA: The American Medical Group Association. They've been around for over thirty years. They report salaries and also include production metrics for multispecialty medical groups. Their surveys are sent to medical groups, and these groups provide the data for the survey results. Again, it costs money to access the survey. This is often the metric that group practices use to determine salaries.

Medscape: There is an annual report named the Medscape Physician Compensation report. This is another report generated from physician surveys. Their report notes that data is compiled from over 19,000 physicians. The thing that sets them apart is that their data is broken down regionally by specialty, gender, race, and age. This can be found for free. Here is the link to the 2018 report: tps://www.medscape.com/slideshow/2018-compensation-overview-6009667

A whole book could be written about the above surveys and how they are used to generate salary numbers, but that is beyond the scope of this book. Do your homework. Get your facts, or the facts will get you.

Merritt Hawkins Review/Actual Value Added

Merritt Hawkins is a national health care professional recruitment company. In 2019, they published the 2019 Physician Inpatient/Outpatient Revenue Survey, which reviews the net revenue generated by physicians for their affiliated hospitals. The survey was sent to CFOs of hospitals across the United States and asked them to estimate how much net revenue was generated by physicians of different specialties. Revenue was reported from hospital admissions, procedures performed at the hospital, tests, treatments ordered, prescriptions written, etc. Revenue generated by referrals to other physicians was excluded.

The average revenue generated for each physician in 2019 was $2,378,727! Every physician should be familiar with the information in Table 1. Granted, there is more to compensation than just salary, but, as we demonstrated in the previous section, there are many forms of value physicians add to a health care system that are not included in these figures. While salary offers will also be based on other factors like location and physician supply, it is vital that physicians understand how valuable they truly are.

Hospitals know and understand this data. While physicians will look at Table 1 and wonder why they are compensated so little compared to the revenue they generate, CFOs will see operating revenue, and CEOs will work to drive the percentages on the right down so that their own bonuses go up! Top executives at several Chicago-area not-for-profit health systems received 37% average yearly raises in 2017. (https://www.modernhealthcare.com/providers/hospital-ceos-get-big-raises-despite-pressure-control-healthcare-costs) Compare that to the yearly increases in salaries for physicians in 2017, where many specialties saw increases in the single digits and pediatrician salaries dropped by 1%! (https://www.medscape.com/slideshow/compensation-2017-urology-6008589#3)

Table 1

Specialty	Avg. Net Revenue	Avg. Salary	% Salary/Revenue
Cardiology (Invasive)	$3,484,375	$590,000	16.9
Cardiology/Non-Inv.	$2,310,000	$427,000	18.5
Cardiovascular Surgery	$3,697,916	$425,000	11.5
Family Practice	$2,111,931	$241,000	11.4
Gastroenterology	$2,965,277	$487,000	16.4
General Surgery	$2,707,317	$350,000	12.9
Hematology/Oncology	$2,855,000	$425,000	14.9
Internal Medicine	$2,675,387	$261,000	9.8
Nephrology	$1,789,062	$272,000	15.2
Neurology	$2,052,884	$301,000	14.7
Neurosurgery	$3,437,500	$687,000	20.0
OB/GYN	$2,024,193	$324,000	16.0
Ophthalmology	$1,440,217	$300,000	20.8
Orthopedic Surgery	$3,286,764	$533,000	16.2
Otolaryngology	$1,937,500	$405,000	20.9
Pediatrics	$1,612,500	$230,000	14.3
Psychiatry	$1,820,512	$261,000	14.3
Pulmonology	$2,361,111	$418,000	17.7
Urology	$2,161,458	$386,000	17.9

A common response when pointing out the data above is, "We can only compensate you based on your professional production." This is not true. It is based on the almost archaic model where physicians own private practices and work in hospitals with whom they have an affiliation. If you are in a private or separate group practice, you cannot be compensated by a hospital for tests and referrals you make to that facility. And, similar to what we noted earlier with respect to referrals, it is not legal to be compensated for each X-ray or lab you order within a system. But, if you are seeking employment from a hospital or health care system, it is reasonable and appropriate to demand a reimbursement package based on the value you add to that system.

Fair Market Value

There is a theoretical limit to your demands. The total value of your compensation package is limited by a never-defined and unclear fair market value, or FMV. Federal anti-kickback and self-referral bans can limit excessive compensation. A hospital that pays far in excess of national averages can be seen as "buying" the tests and referrals that a physician generates. It's a nebulous area of law and one that strikes at the core issue—Is physician behavior modified by these increased salaries? Does a pain management physician order more tests, do more procedures, make more referrals if paid more? My experience has taught me that the exact opposite is true. High base salaries tend to lead to stagnation and decreased work rates, while the private docs I know, on a strictly production model, are engines of medical industry. However, the government, the largest medical payor in the nation, will certainly assume that high salaries induce illicit behaviors and will not be scared to use the full force of the legal system to try and limit payments.

Our solution to the problem of FMV is fairly simple. If all physicians negotiate more aggressively and demand higher reimbursement, those national averages move up. And who can fault someone for getting paid a little better than average?

And one last point: internists—you're getting screwed!

Asking for Information from Local Physicians

A great way to estimate valuation is to speak with other physicians in the geographical area and find out what they are being paid. If you are in residency in Maryland and looking at jobs in rural North Dakota or Iowa, don't talk to your attendings. Instead, do all you can to find out what doctors in Bismarck or Davenport are making. Depending on where and with whom you will be working, this data can be hard to come by. Hospitals may be reticent to share the salaries of other employees, groups may not want to share the details of their top earners, and private practitioners may understate their take-home pay.

Our experience has shown that there are several problems that will arise when trying to obtain and utilize this information. We present them here and give advice to help you overcome them.

Problem 1: Doctors don't openly communicate about salaries and reimbursement. Old-school ideas about the "calling" of medicine and the idea that remuneration is secondary to service still permeate hospital staffs, and getting many doctors to discuss pay is difficult. Physicians may be told that it is against policy to discuss salaries with other providers as well.

Solution 1: Be bold and ask what people are making. If you are interviewing with a large group, ask what the highest salary, median salary, mean salary, and lowest salary are. If they aren't willing to share the data, consider that a red flag. When interviewing with a hospital, ask what others in your specialty are making and how they are being paid.

Consider calling other physicians in the area, even if they work for other institutions, and politely asking if they will share what they are making. The question, respectfully phrased, especially from a resident, may well be answered. When you are asked—be honest and share what you make. If we, as physicians, are more open and honest about reimbursement, it may help us all increase our take-home pay.

Be aware that discussing wages and working conditions is an employee's right under the National Labor Relations Act.

Problem 2: Physicians make erroneous assumptions about their value relative to other physicians.

Many doctors assume that if someone is paid more than them, they are worth less. Physicians may also take offense if others are paid more. This may seem unreal, but we know of physicians who have quit, moved, and left lucrative positions just because they found a colleague was reimbursed at a higher rate.

Elder statesmen may also demand more money because of their experience, and hospitals or practices may try and pay the physician coming out of residency less because of the lack thereof.

Solution 2: Remember that a rising tide lifts all ships. If you find that a colleague received a raise or is being paid more—rejoice. Then, formulate your plan and negotiate your reimbursement upward to match. Remove the emotion and ego from the equation as best you can, and, if necessary, involve a third party in the negotiation to help you avoid making an emotional and financially poor decision.

Understand that pay should be based on education, training, volumes, and competency—not years on the job. If you are coming out of residency and are a capable young physician taking an equal share of call and doing similar volumes, why should you be paid less?

Problem 3: Physicians often have multiple sources of income, and accurate data on true take-home pay can be hard to come by. An employed hospital physician on a salary is pretty straightforward, but a surgeon in a group practice who has ownership of his office building, shares in the local surgery center, and who is receiving reimbursement from the local hospital for taking call may only relate what he is taking home from his practice and leave out the ancillary income.

Solution 3: Be specific in your questions and get it in writing. Ask about every possible revenue stream mentioned by a potential employer and press until you have the answers you need. If the group tells you that you can buy into the surgical center or the office building, find out how much others paid for shares, current property or share valuation, schedules for buy-in, and pay-out for the last several years.

Valuation Summary:

MGMA and other physician compensation outfits are no more than databases of survey results. They are useful as a guidepost but are not definitive. If you are so motivated, spend the time and money to query the databases yourself. At a minimum, find out what inputs were used to calculate the numbers you're being quoted, evaluate the numbers provided in combination with an understanding of your true value, and try and add some local/regional information.

We feel strongly that as you better understand how survey averages are used and realize the true value you add to a health care entity, it will embolden you and weaken negotiation strategies meant to get your labor at a fraction of its actual worth.

Chapter 3: Different Types of Physician Employment Models

Many of our patients think we can do all kinds of surgery. It is not uncommon to have a patient ask Dr. Barton (a general surgeon) to fix their knee, operate on their kidney stones, or manage their sinuses. While we find this fascinating, it's not surprising. Health care specialty practice is complex. The average patient likely only knows generalities about specialty medical training and may only have encountered their PCP or an emergency room physician prior to an appointment with the surgical specialist. Interestingly, we have seen a similar situation with residents' understanding of medical practice models. Many residents may have limited exposure to the world of private or group practice. They will assume that relationships and pay models mirror those with which they are familiar.

There are many types of physician practice models. The names for these models may vary based on group and regional health care system nomenclature, but they often fall into one of the categories listed below. It is imperative that you be familiar with the different practice models and understand the way you will be reimbursed in each in order to effectively negotiate a contract.

Private Practice/Solo Practice

This model of practice is a bit of a dinosaur in medicine. There was a time when physicians would finish training, hang a shingle, and practice medicine. However, the current medical practice environment has become increasingly complex. In the private practice/solo practice model, it's just you and your staff. You can think of this model as the model of silver handcuffs. Physicians sometimes think that if they are their own boss, they can control their schedule. However, expenses never sleep, and unless you find passive sources of income, you must always be working to make this model effective.

We live in an era of Medicare oversight. Medicare sets the rules, and then insurance companies follow. MIPS, MACRA, DRG, CPT, ICD 10, etc. If you don't understand these, then you have a lot to learn, or you shouldn't do private solo practice. If you are committed to this model, we suggest you start learning early and try and find a good practice manager. Just be aware that you will need to be on top of every aspect of your practice, as many physicians have lost millions to the embezzlement of unsupervised practice managers.

If you are considering the private practice model but plan to purchase a practice that is already in place, you will need to negotiate the purchase of the practice. This topic is beyond the scope of this book. If you are interested in pursuing either the creation or purchase of a solo practice, here are some key points you should consider:

1. How are coding and billing set up, or how will it be set up?

2. Do you have any insurance contracts established? Will you have any help in negotiating your rates with local insurances? This is HUGE. If you are doing this alone, the chances of your success are low.

3. What does the payer mix look like?

4. If established, how long are the contracts with insurance companies in effect? How good are these insurance contracts, and are they transferrable with the practice?

5. Who manages the office, or who will? (The office manager serves multiple roles in these practices, and if you're purchasing an established practice and the office manager doesn't come with the package, just run). Can you trust this person, and do you have the financial background to detect embezzlement if it is occurring?

6. Can you look at a year's worth of balance sheets or projections to determine the seasonal variation in the practice?

7. What is or what will be the debt to income ratio?

8. What are the demographics of the patient population?

9. Which EMR will you use, and who will provide IT support? (It is unrealistic to provide Medicare, and therefore industry-standard complaint care without an IT platform)

10. How old are and how much exists in accounts receivable?

11. What facilities and equipment will you need? How will you pay for them? Can you secure the loans that may be needed to get things up and running?

12. Are you prepared for a several-month lag between rendering services and reimbursement?

13. Are there competing medical interests in the area? If you will be dependent on referrals, can you guarantee they will occur? Big Health Care is notorious for leaning on their physicians to refer to other providers in the same system—beware.

There is one type of private/solo practice model that can be less complex than that noted above. These are practices that are straight fee for service, meaning that the providers don't accept Medicare or private insurance. In this model, a patient walks in the door and pays cash for a service. This model is often used in cosmetic practices and urgent care but, in our experience, is not an option for many specialties and would be difficult to implement for most.

If, after careful consideration, you are convinced that private solo practice is your future, find a mentor, an office manager, an accountant, an attorney, and a therapist. Then, you can proceed.

Solo Practice/Hospital Income Guarantee

This is a hybrid model. The basic premise is that you are employed by the hospital but practice by yourself. The hospital supports your practice, and you work with the hospital as a team. This joint venture is set up in several different ways. Here is the most common scenario we have seen:

The hospital provides you with office space, staffing, and coding/billing. You provide the labor. As a provider, you are guaranteed a set income (hence the term income guarantee). Let's pick a number of $350,000. As long as you meet the minimum guidelines required for work as outlined in the contract, you'll make $350,000 a year. If you want to make more money, you have to cover your salary and the expenses for items/services the hospital provides. Using the example above with a salary of $350,000, and assuming that it costs $100,000 to run the practice, you would need to generate $450,000 in net revenue, after which the excess would be split between you and the hospital in a manner decided upon in your contract.

This is not a bad model for lucrative practices. However, it can be a punitive model for rural areas or for specialty practices that are not high revenue-generating. It is also easy to get taken advantage of in this model. Here are a few quick examples:

Let's say you are a surgeon. Your base is the $350,000 mentioned above. Your practice generates $500,000 in net revenue a year minus the extra $100,000 in practice expenses that leaves $50,000 left for you and the hospital to split as bonus money. But the hospital tells you that they need to charge you a bit extra to do some upgrades on your clinic space. Or they tell you that the EMR is outdated and must be replaced. Before you know it, that $50,000 is whittled down or disappears entirely.

Alternatively, they may offer you shared staff, meaning your practice staff is shared with other clinic providers in the same system. Now, *they* are saving expenses, but *you* still have the same overhead. In the process, your practice efficiency declines, and it makes less revenue. Or, what if coding and billing isn't efficient and your practice cannot make the revenue to cover baseline expenses? Then, the hospital comes to you and says they are losing money on your practice. They say they need to decrease your salary because of this. Before you know it, you're making less.

Unfortunately, this happens all the time. The only way to combat this is to have contractual protection!

Here are several important questions for those considering an income guarantee model:

1. What are your fixed costs? What is the base amount charged by the hospital for your practice? What items and services are included in these costs?
2. What are the variable costs? These are expenses that can be added by the hospital to the base cost. Do they charge you a flat fee for coding and billing? Do they charge you a percentage of collections? Does staffing change costs?
3. What do you have control over? Specifically, can you control who works in the office with you? Having a bad staff member can decimate you and your business. Do you have any say over staffing?
4. How does the hospital calculate your revenue? Hospitals can calculate this from gross receipts, insurance payments, patient collections, accounts receivable (yes, they can count "potential" money in your accounts receivable as revenue), and so forth. How do these variables add to your revenue?
5. What is your base income, and will this ever decrease or increase?
6. What is the term of the guarantee?
7. How do you get out of the guarantee? Meaning, if you make enough to pay off all the hospital expenses, can you leave the agreement? Or, if it's obvious you'll never cover the hospital's expenses for your practice, do you have options?
8. Can the hospital refer you to another physician who is currently employed under this model? This may be the most important thing to ask. Learn from others!

Multispecialty and Single Specialty Group Practice

Medical group practices use complex revenue models, and there are as many variations as there are words in this book. Payment models are often based on fee-for-service (you eat what you kill) with some supplements to income from lab, radiology, drug administration, rents, and other sources of clinic-owned income. Deductions to salary will include malpractice, health insurance, and any retirement plans you choose to use. You will also likely be charged for rent, supplies, coding/billing, staffing, and may even be asked/told that you are contributing portions of projected income for costs accrued by the whole group (such as management, loans, building expenses, consultants, etc). Some physicians (partners) may be reimbursed more than incoming physicians based on ownership of assets, with incoming doctors expected to "buy in" before receiving equivalent payments.

If you are considering a group like this, we have a few suggestions:

1. Ask for their specific payment model and have it reviewed by your accountant. (Those we have seen are inordinately complex, and even some accountants go cross-eyed trying to decipher them.)

2. Ask to see the payment model calculations for the last several months for the top, median, and bottom producers in the clinic. (We know of a full-time urologist whose total reimbursement after paying for all the clinic costs was under $10 one month! Understand the limits of your reimbursement.)

3. Make sure ownership/partnership terms are clearly delineated and guaranteed. You don't want to be making the partners money by working your buns off for two to three years only to discover that the partnership you were promised is now not available or exorbitantly priced. In general, we would recommend you consider buy-in for physical facilities and tangible assets but refuse buy into the practice.

4. Be honest with yourself about how much you want to work and are willing to produce. That top producer you asked about might be working eighty hours a week.

5. Understand that individuals in your same specialty in your same clinic are your competition, not your colleagues. Don't expect

any of them to sacrifice business and money to keep you adequately reimbursed.

6. Understand that when you go on vacation, your expenses don't. As in private practice, if you take a week off, you will not only lose the reimbursement for all the work you would have done but will also still be paying rent, staffing, insurance, etc.

Hospital Employed Production Model

In this model of employment, you will be paid for your professional production based on either collections or predetermined production units such as RVUs. In the former model, there is often a calculation that deducts anticipated expenses from cash received, whereas, with the latter, the costs are typically anticipated and calculated into the RVU multiplier. To illustrate, we will use two *very* simplistic examples.

A. You generate $3 million in billing, the hospital collects $600,000, and after deducting anticipated expenses of $200,000, your take-home pay is $400,000. This is paid out as a base salary of $20,000 per month ($240,000/year) with the remaining $160,000 coming as a bonus at the end of your financial/contract year.

B. Your contract specifies an RVU multiplier of $42/RVU. Every CPT code you generate is assigned an RVU value based on values predetermined by CMS (Centers for Medicare & Medicaid Services). At the end of the year, you generated 8,473 RVUs and earned $355,866. You had been receiving $20,000 per month ($240,000/year), and the remaining $115,866 is paid as a bonus at the end of your financial/contract year.

At the end of each year, base salary may be moved up or down based on past performance and projections for the upcoming year. Variations and complexities to these formulae exist, but the basic ideal is still fee-for-service. Other incentive payments may be incorporated in this model and are addressed in the combined (Salary + Incentive) model later in this chapter.

If you plan to work for a hospital on a production model, these are our suggestions:

1. Be realistic about production goals, and how much/hard you want to work. We know docs who generate 17,000 RVUs per year, but they don't do much else outside of work.

2. If possible, consider RVU-based models. Cash collection models may look enticing, but coding and billing are fickle and the facility's failure to collect leaves you holding the bag. This is especially true if you have high rates of nonpaying patients.

3. If you are getting paid on receipts/collections, ask for a breakdown of coverage in the area and be aware of the percentages of nonpaying patients and those with poorly paying plans such as Medicaid.

4. As always, ask for data (receipts, RVUs, RVU multipliers) for others at the facility, especially those in the same specialty.

5. Negotiate your RVU multiplier aggressively! A dollar or two more per RVU can have significant implications on your paycheck.

6. Understand that individuals in your same specialty at your hospital are your competition, not your colleagues. Don't expect any of them to sacrifice business and money to keep you adequately reimbursed.

7. Be careful with the base salary. If you are being compensated more than you are producing, you will have to pay it back—often as deductions from future production.

8. Remember that **total compensation must be capped** to decrease the risk of fair-market value violations. As such, highly productive physicians may need to accept lower pay per work unit than others—providing a perverse counter-incentive to excess production.

Hospital Employed Salaried Position (W-2 Income)

You negotiate a yearly salary, sign the deal, go to work, see patients, you get a paycheck deposited in your account every two weeks. Expenses, coding, billing, and malpractice insurance are all taken care of, and you can focus on taking care of patients. Your benefits package includes paid CME, 401(k), and health and disability insurance. You have paid vacation, and even when you are gone, the paychecks land with regularity.

This is perhaps the simplest payment model, but there are still some areas to watch out for. Here are our recommendations:

1. Talk to other employed physicians and find out how much they are pushed to produce. In this model, the facility—not you—makes more money when you work hard, and they will often try and press more and more out of you.

2. Negotiate salary aggressively. You won't be able to make more with sweat and blood, so ask for what you want up front.

3. Negotiate vacation aggressively. Perhaps the biggest benefit to this model is the ability to take real time away without impacting your bottom line, so get as much time as you can.

4. Scrutinize call requirements carefully. A salaried position with no coverage when you're gone or constant ER call responsibilities can make you feel like a slave.

5. Consider the tax implications of this type of position. Most employed/salaried positions will provide W-2 income, so you will be paying the highest possible tax rates. Your cell phone, travel, and other expenses will not be deductible.

Hospital Employed Blended (Salary + Incentive Bonus)

In this model, you have a guaranteed floor for your salary. Like the pure salary model above, your expenses are typically covered and your benefits guaranteed. Your income will be constant and stable for most of the year, but there are opportunities to increase your take-home pay with extra work or other incentives. As in the production models, you will have cash receipt or RVU targets that, if exceeded, will be paid through to you as a bonus.

Here's an example. If you negotiated a salary of $400,000 as a guaranteed base salary and also negotiated a base RVU rate of $45/RVU, then the first 8,888 RVUs (400,000/45) generated will offer you no benefit. But, if you exceeded this target and generated 9,500 RVUs in the fiscal year, you would get a nice bonus of $27,500 at the end of the year. If, on the other hand, you were slower than expected and generated only 7,900 RVUs, you would still receive the $400,000 per year guaranteed.

Production targets like collections, charges, visits, or RVUs are the most common in these types of contracts, but physician pay can also be based on value or quality incentives, such as outcomes (hospital readmissions, post-op infections, BP target successes), patient satisfaction, process measures (charting, screening measure compliance like mammograms), or citizenship (attending meetings or sitting on committees). Incentives may be incremental or tiered (e.g., bonus is only achieved after every 500 extra RVUs) and are often included in contracts to maximize organizational profits.

If you choose this model, we offer the following suggestions:

1. Aggressively negotiate your base salary. A high base salary can put the burden of marketing, patient recruitment, and even coding/billing on your employer. And, a high base salary makes your vacations less worrisome.

2. Realize that, in this model, your vacation days may rob you of bonus money. We know physicians in this model who have a much harder time taking vacation because they are aware of the effect on the year-end bonus.

3. Negotiate your RVU multiplier aggressively! A dollar or two more per RVU can have significant implications on your paycheck.

4. Ask to see production numbers and bonus payments for others in your specialty for several years. Some facilities and systems will move the production requirements/RVU goals on providers, making it harder and harder to earn bonuses. Make sure bonus requirements are clearly outlined in your contract and that the hospital can't change them unilaterally. Remember that if production bonuses are unattainable, they are worthless.

5. Be honest with yourself about how much you're willing to work and how much you're likely to generate. Ask colleagues about hours worked and RVUs generated.

6. Don't bank on the bonuses. Hospitals know what you're likely to produce and are notorious for dangling that carrot just beyond your reach.

7. As with the salaried position, you must scrutinize call and tax implications carefully.

8. Remember that **total compensation may be capped** to decrease the risk of fair-market value violations. As such, highly productive physicians may need to accept lower pay per work unit than others—providing a perverse counter-incentive to excess production.

Academic Position

Working in academic medicine can both complicate and simplify your reimbursement. Academic positions may have affiliations with private hospitals, state-run community hospitals, federally run hospitals (VA), and major academic institutions. These positions typically require clinical work, teaching medical students/residents/other providers in training, administrative work, and research. So, how, then, is one reimbursed? Will you be paid for only your clinical work? If you land a huge grant, does some of that money come to you? Will you be paid separately by the associated hospitals, or will all money flow through the parent institution?

We all owe our training to academic medicine and are products of the system. Almost all physicians, therefore, have some familiarity with its convoluted landscape. We also know that there is something noble in teaching and conducting meaningful clinical research and that many who pursue academic careers find motivation in benefits outside financial remuneration such as titles and status or in true altruism. This being said, you must remember that both ego and altruism can be exploited. And, you must therefore be careful to as you evaluate and negotiate your position. You should always know who signs your checks.

If working in the ivory tower of academic medicine is what you want, here are some points to consider:

1. Find out what entities you will be working for. As mentioned above, you need to delineate who your employers are. Are you an employee of the hospital, the department, or the institute of higher learning affiliated with the residency program? Ask how each institution at which you will be working contributes to your salary.

2. Realize that, as you negotiate with a department chair, they may only be a liaison for another entity.

3. Realize that, in this model, there may be little room for salary negotiation. If everyone in the department is getting paid the same amount, you're not likely to get any more.

4. With salary negotiations often difficult or impossible, you should focus heavily on negotiating other details of the contract such as call, administrative responsibilities, research, etc.

5. Ask for copies of policies on grant money and make sure you understand how the work you do securing funding will impact your bottom line and how such money will be distributed.

6. Make sure your workload is defined very specifically. Sometimes junior faculty become the dumping ground for the work of tenured faculty. Think of yourself as joining a group practice where your new group may be the whole department. Don't accept extra work unless there are clearly attached financial or professional benefits.

7. If you plan to advance in academic medicine, make sure the pathway and expectations are clearly defined. Typically, progression starts with an assistant professorship and progresses as follows: Assistant-Associate-Full-Endowed-Distinguished-Administrative-Emeritis. Trust us. This is a food chain. Progression to full professor requires that you hit certain milestones that may include teaching, publication, clinical volumes, and other metrics. These milestones need to be spelled out. Arbitrary progression rules could place you at the mercy of others. Not progressing could cost you money, lifestyle, and job security. Request a clear path to advancement in your contract.

8. Make sure the allocation of your time is very clearly spelled out. It is easy for teaching and clinical duties to encroach on research. It's even easier for clinical work to encroach on teaching. Before you realize what's happening, you could become the faculty member that works more than the residents! Finding the right balance in an academic position is a challenge. One rule of thumb is to have an administrative day spelled out in your contract and then protect it with your life. The same principle applies to research. Without dedicated time to work on research, it will only eat up your personal time. Have your responsibilities clearly defined and then have them delineated so that you have time to perform all the necessary tasks of your profession.

9. Remember that the world of academic medicine is small. Understand that your first job may be the launching pad to the position at the well-respected institution of which you've always dreamed. Because academics tend to jump around chasing the next rung on the moving professional ladder, you need to find out about contract termination. It is perceived as a sensitive subject that is difficult to bring up; however, addressing this issue is vital when you negotiate an academic contract.

10. Talk to the junior faculty wherever you're interviewing. Talk to the residents. Have these conversations without oversight from any department personnel. You can learn a lot by observation.

Contracted Individual or Group Practices

In this model, the physician or group of physicians have a contract with a hospital or health care system to provide services. When the services are rendered, they are reimbursed. In this model, the physician or group is its own business entity, and payments will be reported on a 1099. The receiving entity will be responsible for employment taxes and providing all other benefits such as retirement, vehicles, insurance, etc.

As an example: A large anesthesia group has a contract to provide services to a multihospital system. It recruits you to join the group, and you set up your own LLC. The group schedules you to work at a facility; you provide anesthesia services all day and then submit your work to the group, which then bills the hospital system. The money is paid to the group, which takes a portion to provide services to you on which you have agreed (malpractice and health insurance), and the rest comes to your business as income. As an LLC, you can then deduct expenses accrued in providing services.

If this model is an option, consider the following:

1. Consider this option strongly if you have benefits provided in another way. If a spouse's employer pays for health insurance and strong retirement funding, this model may allow you to turn benefit costs into take-home pay.
2. You will need a good accountant to help with running the business. Quarterly tax payments, assuring appropriate deductions, retirement plan setup, and more will now fall on your shoulders.
3. Understand partnership requirements because groups like this may have tiers of ownership/partnership that can limit initial pay. Make sure you know how and when advancement in the company will take place.
4. Negotiate the terms of service carefully and focus on the duration of the contract. A hospital may want to terminate

your service contract if they find a newly minted resident willing to work as an employee for half as much.

You may encounter models of practice not covered in this section. If you do, demand data, review carefully, involve your accountant and attorney, and negotiate like your life depends on it.

Chapter 4: More Than Salary: Other Monetary Considerations

Up to this point, we have really focused on salary as the primary negotiation goal. We feel that it should be the main point of consideration, as it can significantly impact your quality of life, and loss of salary can really add up over years in a position. However, there are many other financial pieces to your employment package that should be considered, and that can be reasons for taking or leaving a new position.

Signing Bonuses

Physicians of in-demand specialties can expect to be offered a lump sum that is payable at the time a contract is signed or at the time work commences. We have seen bonuses ranging from $3,000 to $100,000 offered to physicians to fill needed voids. These payments are often used as financial incentives (or disincentive) to lure physicians in or prevent physicians from leaving. In short, they give you big money up front, you promise to stay for a certain number of years, and if you leave early, you have to pay them back.

We have seen a few primary forms of these bonuses.

In the first scenario, bonuses are paid to the physician as a lump sum payment and have immediate tax implications. That is to say, if you get $25,000, your income statement for the year will include that full amount, which will be subject to income taxes. In this model, there are typically penalties for early departure. If you leave before 36 months of work, you will have to pay (1/36 x number of months early that you are leaving x bonus amount) as a penalty.

Another model will provide the signing bonus as a "loan." You receive all the money up front, and a percentage is forgiven for each year you stay in the job. In this model, you have no tax implications up front but will have to pay taxes on the amount forgiven + interest accrued on that amount in the year that the portion of the loan is forgiven. So, if you get a $10,000 signing bonus forgiven at 25% each year, you'll have to pay taxes on $2,500 (plus interest—don't forget that part) each of the following four years. And if you leave in 3 years, 25% will be subject to payback upon your exit.

A few pointers when negotiating or accepting a signing bonus:

1. Make sure you like the place before you lock yourself in. Review Dr. Barton's story from the start of this book if you need data on how often physicians leave their first job. You really don't want to be stuck in a bad position because you can't afford to leave.

2. Remember that signing bonuses are short-term and salary is long. Don't give up $25,000 per year of salary for an extra $25,000 signing bonus. Your signing bonus will not pay you more over the next 10 years you work, but that higher pay rate sure might.

3. Consider the tax implications of the sign-on bonus carefully and consult with your accountant, financial advisor, or other tax professional. You may want to keep a significant portion of the bonus in a liquid account in case the taxes are more than you anticipated.

4. Review the payback stipulations carefully. Punitive conditions for payback are possible. You don't want to work 35 months of a 36-month contract, leave early, and find that you owe the entire signing bonus.

5. Make sure you know your interest rate. If your signing bonus is considered a loan, the interest rate will affect how much you pay in taxes each year. Again, consult with your accountant and financial advisor to make sure you are paying reasonable rates.

Residency Stipends

Health care companies, practices, and hospitals know that you're starving. Okay, you have enough to eat, but you're probably in your 30s, have a mountain of debt, may have a family, and are living off a resident's fixed income. So, the promise of a few thousand dollars a month for the last twelve months of residency can seem like a godsend. That is exactly what a residency stipend is: prepayment, often monthly, for a period of time prior to the completion of your residency and commencement of work. It is, in effect, a signing bonus, and all of the points above should be considered. We would advise you to do the math and calculate the total dollar amount of any offered stipend. Don't accept less tomorrow for a morsel today.

Loan Repayment

Medical student loan debt is increasing faster than American BMIs. The weight of that debt can be suffocating and can impact your finances for decades. Potential employers understand this and will offer to make payments directly to your loans as part of your employment package. In addition to salary and signing bonuses, they may offer $X,000 per year toward student loan repayment for a period of 2-3 years.

A few things to consider here:

1. Anything you receive will count as income. If the hospital you are joining sends $30,000 to your student loan debt, you will have to pay taxes on $30,000 of income, thereby lowering your take-home pay by the amount of excess tax paid. Consider tax implications carefully and consult with your accountant.
2. Realize that employers use this incentive to lower salary/reimbursement. Student loan repayment of $30,000 yearly for three years is much cheaper than a $30,000 extra salary x 30 years.

In the end, we suggest you focus your efforts on maximizing your take-home pay. You can then use the extra money to pay off loans if you want, but the decision remains in your hands.

CME Money

Many employed positions will give you a CME (Continuing Medical Education) stipend. A few thousand dollars a year is not uncommon. This money is used to pay for testing, courses, airfare, rental cars, hotels, or any other costs you incur while getting the CME you need to maintain licensure and certification. It isn't a huge concern, and hospitals may pay the same amount to every physician in their system, but be aware that, like everything else, it is negotiable. If you live and work in a remote area, costs for travel will be much higher. Ask for what you need.

Pensions and Retirement Accounts

If you haven't figured it out yet, we don't trust health care companies to do what is best for physicians. And that includes when they tell you that they are going to take some of your money, invest it for you, and then provide you with that money when you retire. There are many examples of strong, stable, bedrock companies whose pension plans failed. For that reason, we would advise that you be very cautious when planning on the promises of even the biggest health care companies to provide you with a pension. We feel that, like the process of finding a job and negotiating a deal, it's best when you retain control.

In brief, pensions and retirement plans are forms of delayed compensation. It is money that you or your employer puts away every year that you work, with the promise that upon retirement, you will receive a benefit. There are several ways these plans can be funded (employee or employer) and several ways that the benefits can be paid back (defined benefit vs. defined contribution.). Be aware that for many private practice/group practice models, you are the employee and employer, and all contributions to a retirement plan will come directly out of the income you generate. Plans may also be subject to vesting periods and delays in funding, and we would encourage you to find out the details of the retirement vehicles that your potential employer is offering and review them with your accountant and financial advisor.

In our experience, due to the complexity of administering these plans, there is very little room to change the way they are run or amounts of employer contribution in negotiation. Therefore, your best bet is to do your homework, employ the aid of professionals to understand the offered plans, and select employment with the best plans you can find. Once you sign a contract, continue to consult with your advisors as you move through enrollment.

Health, Life and Disability Insurance

Almost every position we know comes with a health insurance plan. Just like with the retirement plans above, the provision of health insurance is typically defined by what the group or hospital has chosen, and there is very little room for negotiation. It is still worth your time to make sure that you understand the health, vision, and dental benefits provided. When you're at that interview lunch with other docs and their spouses, ask if they have a family and what they think of their health plan. You'll likely find out more from these responses than from those of the HR representative.

Flexible spending accounts (FSA) and health savings accounts (HSA) are also frequently offered tax-advantaged plans. FSAs allow you to set apart a small portion of your income pre-tax to cover qualified medical expenses every year. Funds may or may not be allowed to roll over into a new year if unused. HSAs allow you to save pre-tax dollars in an account that can be invested and then used for medical expenses or nonmedical expenses with some possible attached penalties. HSAs require you to be enrolled in a high-deductible health insurance plan and may not be best for some individuals or families. The nuances of these plans are beyond the scope of this book. Discuss the plans with your future employer, family, and accountant before you decide what is best for you.

Some benefit plans will also include life insurance. The amount of life insurance is often minimal (one year of salary or so), with the potential to buy significantly increased coverage if you so desire. In our experience, the rates offered by third-party insurance providers are often better than rates offered through your employer. The insurance offered and rates are also typically not negotiable. As such, we would recommend you negotiate more pay and shop around to find the best life insurance package you can.

Disability insurance is a trickier subject, and we have seen significant differences in how disability is offered. As a high-income earner, a few months away from your job can put a dent in your finances, and a life-altering injury or illness could be devastating. You want to ask about both short-term and long-term disability and make sure you know exactly how each is provided and the amounts covered.

Short-term disability will often kick in fairly soon after the injury or illness and cover thirty to ninety days of expenses. Some employers will provide sick leave instead of short-term disability, and others will have no short-term plan at all. Make sure you know what is covered, the dates after injury or illness when coverage starts, and whether or not you'll be required to use your vacation days prior to use of disability or sick leave. If you haven't built up a sufficient emergency fund, consider paying for some short-term coverage through a third party if none is available to you.

Long-term disability similarly is often offered at a price but may not be offered at all. As with short-term coverage, make sure you know how much you will be paid when your long-term coverage starts and for how long. Make sure that your coverage will pay you if you are not able to do the work you trained to do "same specialty coverage" and won't require you to repeat a residency in another specialty.

Remember that the amount of disability insurance coverage you have will need to cover your expenses and potentially allow you to save for retirement as well. If you're expecting a sizable inheritance from Grandpa Warbucks or if you know that your parents will come to your rescue, this may not be a concern. But we have seen doctors incapacitated due to illness who had insufficient long-term disability, and their families suffered greatly due to the lack thereof. In general, we would recommend that you max out your long-term disability and consider the addition of third-party coverage if you have dependents. As with all benefits plans, the terms of disability coverage may not be negotiable, but the presence of short- and long-term coverage and the ability to buy up that coverage should not be overlooked.

Dues and Licenses

A medical license isn't cheap. When you decide on a job, it's not unusual to find out that the State Board of Medicine wants $65 for a background check, $200 for the application, and another $300 every year. The DEA now demands $731 for a 3-year license. Your specialty board group kindly requests $200 a year after you pay $2,000 for the test they require you to pass. And the national association you join is $100 a year, with the regional section lifting another $75 yearly from your wallet.

With that in mind, make sure you know who is going to pay for all that. Many practices will cover state and DEA licensure, but others may expect you to deduct those costs from your CME budget. If it isn't stipulated, ask for these costs to be covered. If you're expected to cover the costs from CME funds, make sure they are adequate for all the bills and a conference or two as well.

Moving Expenses

Ah, the good ol' days when moving expenses were tax-deductible. Prior to 2018, many moving expenses were deductible if you were moving a certain distance because of a job change. In the past scenario, if the hospital paid the moving company $15,000 to box your stuff and cart it across the country and then sent you a 1099 tax form, you could deduct much or all of that $15,000 from your taxes. But alas, no more! Changes to tax law have made it so that any reimbursement for moving expenses is taxable income, subject to income and employment taxes and any other required withholdings (exceptions apply for military members).

Under the old system, having moving expenses paid was a great benefit, especially for the cash-strapped resident. And still, having moving expenses covered may be the only way to get your junk from point A to point B. Just be aware that higher moving costs (hiring a moving company, having cars shipped, flying to your destination) may mean more of your arduously negotiated and hard-earned salary going to Uncle Sam.

Employers know this but are also aware of the financial straits in which many residents find themselves. They will proudly list "Moving Allowance of $15,000" on their job offer but are unlikely to advise of the tax consequences. Whatever you do, work to keep your moving costs down. You may even want to research moving expenses, negotiate the expected cost into your signing bonus, and then move yourself using the cheapest way possible, thereby profiting if you come in under budget.

Creative Monetary Demands

When the NFL's leading rusher is negotiating his new contract, you can bet that his agent is working on getting him a gold-plated Ferrari with his jersey number stitched in the seat leather. If Miles Finch is coming to your publishing firm, he's going to need a black limo with the internal temp at exactly 71 degrees. So, if the hospital or clinic where you are headed really needs you and you have some financial request that will make the move feasible, consider placing it on the negotiation table.

We know of individuals in the oil industry who have had their old homes purchased by a new employer to facilitate a move. We've heard of individuals receiving housing allowances or tuition assistance. An extra trip out to your prospective new hometown to allow you, your spouse, or older children to look for housing and scout out schools would be eminently reasonable. Historically, physicians haven't asked for or received any of these things. But past failures need not persist. The key here will be having sound reasons for your demands and communicating them effectively.

Chapter 5: More Than Money: Lifestyle Considerations

If there is one piece of advice that we would give to every medical student trying to choose a field of medicine, it would be to consider more carefully your future lifestyle. Many medical specialties are intellectually stimulating, provide opportunities to serve those in need, pay reasonably well, and are even kinda cool and sexy. But cool, sexy, financially rewarding, and stimulating won't keep you practicing if you feel overworked, exhausted, anxious, or depressed. Work/life balance is increasingly difficult to find, and high rates of physician burnout and suicide are concerning to all of us who value colleagues, health, and health care.

As with all of the monetary considerations discussed up to this point, you cannot and must not assume that the clinics, hospitals, and other employers you will be working for will prioritize your lifestyle and health. The recruiter will tell you about all of the fabulous activities available in the area (the lake is 15 minutes away, the major city nearby has NFL and NBA franchises, the local orchestra does a series of outdoor concerts, etc.), and you will be assured that the doctors in your group enjoy ample opportunities for travel and relaxation. But, when the hospital has no call coverage because another doctor in your specialty left town, they often won't think twice about beating you over the head with your own sense of duty and a poorly worded contract that requires you to take call and cover the ER twenty days a month. You must negotiate your vacation, call, and time away from clinical responsibilities as fiercely or more fiercely than your salary.

Vacation

Time away from your practice can be a lifesaver. Vacation isn't the only answer to the complex problem of burnout, but from our experience, it can help immeasurably. Some physicians live and breathe medicine—and a night away from the hospital means "they missed out on a cool case." But most of us, the sane ones, at least, will want to spend some time alone or with family and friends completely free from the pressures of practice and call.

So how much vacation time is "standard"? That is one fantastic and loaded question. The answer to that question will vary greatly depending on your definition of vacation. Do you mean paid time off or time away from your practice?

Paid Time Off vs. Time Away

Paid Time Off: For the strictly salaried employee with 6 weeks of vacation and CME time per year, vacation is truly vacation. If you take 3 weeks off for that dream vacation to Europe, you won't notice any difference in your paychecks or on your W-2 at the end of the year. Your vacation days are accumulated as you work. As an example: You may earn ~0.56 vacation days for each week worked for a total of 30 vacation days per year (0.56 x 52). You can often use the vacation before it is truly earned, with the caveat that if you quit before earning those days, you would have to pay your employer back. Vacation days in this scenario are often use 'em or lose 'em. So, if you take only 25 days off and are due 30, you lose five days when the year resets.

The number of days of contracted vacation can vary widely. If you're a radiologist or pathologist, you may have 10 or 12 weeks a year. If you're a surgeon working for a big health care conglomerate, 5 weeks might be all you get. Oh, and they're going to need you to cover the weekend before you leave.

If you are going to work in a strictly salaried position, negotiate aggressively for your vacation days and then guard them ferociously.

Be aware that you'll often be met with false anchors: "We offer five weeks to everyone, and we just can't do any more than that." You may also face the plying of your better qualities to limit your use of those days: "Dr. Smith is gone, and if you take your last week of vacation, we won't have any coverage for the ER."

Time Away: For the physician in private practice, group practice, or employed position with a production-based contract, time away is a much more nebulous concept.

If you've ever read *Rich Dad, Poor Dad* by Robert Kyosaki, you'll know the difference between a businessman and one who is self-employed. The businessman provides capital (both financial and intellectual) and builds a business machine that continues to run, even when he is not there pressing the buttons and pulling the levers. The self-employed individual is the main lever-puller, and when he stops or takes a break, the business machine screeches to a halt.

If you are in production-linked practice, you will quickly learn that it is not the cost of the vacation that gets you, but the cost of leaving your office building and employees behind while you take the economic engine of the office (YOU!) out for a walk on the beach. The rent is still due, the lights are still on, and support staff will still be working.

In these models, you may also find that because of monthly fixed costs (rent, staffing, power, gas, internet, EMR, etc.), the real valuable work, that which provides the take-home pay you and your family rely upon, is done in the last week of the month. And when you take a vacation or days away, you lose the profitable portion of the month's work. The bills still get paid. The doctor...not so much.

Dr. Van Bibber: *"When I interviewed for my first job, I asked about vacation. I was assured, with no additional explanation, that I could take "whatever time off I wanted." That sounded great until I entered practice and realized that taking even a day or two off could completely sink my monthly production and lower my take-home pay considerably. My former partner, still working in that same practice, told me he was taking his week of vacation over the end of January* and into February so that the days off were split across two different months. It was far too expensive to take a full week off any given month!"

CME Time

Every state medical board or specialty board is going to want to make sure you spend as much money and time as possible jumping through meaningless CME hoops. Many employers know this and will provide additional time away for the fulfillment of CME requirements. For the purposes of contracting, just remember that CME time is essentially vacation time with a purpose. As such, all of the points for vacation time above apply. If you're salaried, you'll be able to take time without changes to compensation. If you're on a production pay model, you'll pay for CME twice!

Call

Whether you're talking about call for the ER, call for colleagues, or just call for your own patients, time on-call is a voracious life leach that you must evaluate carefully when negotiating your contract. In our experience, contract sections governing call expectations are often very vague and nebulous, and efforts to better define call are often met with some resistance. Contracts might say you are required to take "an equal share" of call, "standard call," or "call to be determined by your specialty." Such vague terms often benefit employers, as "an equal share" can change dramatically when your group of four loses two partners!

ER call can also be left out of your contract entirely and come as a requirement for admitting privileges at hospitals in your area. It is imperative that you delineate the different types of call and that you set limits to protect yourself. It is also increasingly common for certain specialties to be reimbursed for taking call—another area where you will want to negotiate aggressively.

Emergency Room/Hospital Call

Hospital employees will often be expected to take some ER or hospital call as part of their contract. Self-employed or group-employed physicians may not have any set call requirements other than those specified by the bylaws of hospitals to which they admit patients. If there are several physicians of a specialty in the area, whether in one group or more, call may be negotiated with these individuals.

Hospital bylaws will often require that you be available and respond to call within a certain amount of time, depending on your specialty. These shifts are often measured or meted out in 24-hour blocks, meaning that a day of call also means a night of call. And if you are a modern-day resident, used to turning into a pumpkin and going home to catch a few Zs after a night of call, the full day in the office or operating room that follows that busy night of emergency procedures can be a real kick in the teeth. If call is busy, 5 days a month can be devastating to your health, and even if call is not busy, it can prevent you from leaving town, participating in recreational activities, or even going out for drinks with friends.

We urge you not to downplay the impact ER call will have on your life. When reviewing your contract and evaluating any position consider the following with regard to inpatient and ER call:

1. Set clearly defined call limits. (i.e., Physician will not be required to take more than X days/calendar month.) The limit will vary considerably by specialty, as seven days of call/month for an orthopedic surgeon will likely generate ten times more calls than an entire year of dermatology call. You may also want to define how many weekday vs. weekends are required. Do not accept a position based on nebulous call language or on a promise that it will get figured out, as the "figuring-out" will often come with pressure applied on the physician to cover more than they really want.

2. Make sure call shifts are clearly defined and time limits specified. When does call start? When does it end? How is handoff taken care of? What are call shifts for weekends? If it isn't spelled out, you can assume that the answer will not be to your benefit.
3. If in a specialty where backup call is required, apply steps 1 and 2 above to backup call as well.
4. Negotiate call pay aggressively, i.e., "For any call shift over 7 per month, physician will be reimbursed at a rate of $3000 per 24-hour call." Or, if you are not a hospital employee, "Each 24-hour ER/inpatient call shift for Hospital X will be reimbursed at a rate of $3000 per 24-hour period."
5. Realize that call reimbursement can be guaranteed money whereas production bonuses can be difficult to reach. Increasing call pay and call amounts can dramatically increase your "base" pay, allowing you to decrease your workload in the clinic if you so choose.
6. Get copies of bylaws for any hospitals where you will be practicing and review call expectations. Don't find out after taking the job with the local clinic that admitting privileges require an "equal share of call" or some other such nonsense.
7. Discuss call expectations with partners or competitors in the area. If the four crusty old surgeons in the area have always taken call for free and feel that that is the way things should be, you are unlikely to get paid.
8. Check with the practice accountant or hospital accountant to make sure call is reimbursed at the rates you're being quoted. Trust but verify!
9. Don't feel compelled to take more call than you are comfortable taking. Just because the ER is uncovered isn't a reason for you to work more days and nights for free.

10. If possible, find out the volumes of inpatient and ER calls by specialty and evaluate your anticipated workload.
11. Make sure you know who is to cover in the event of your absence. If you take three weeks off for vacation in July and you've only taken three of your required seven days of monthly call before you leave, what happens with call? Some hospitals may require that YOU hire a locums to cover your call if you don't meet your obligations.

Practice Coverage and Patient Phone Calls

A hospital recruiter once told a client of ours that call at their facility was ten days per month. He was to be the only practitioner in his specialty in the community. With our prodding, he asked how phone calls and other questions from the local community were handled and soon found out that he would be solely responsible for any patient phone calls or clinical questions if he was in town. So, in reality, there were ten days of ER call PLUS thirty to thirty-one days of being tied to his cell phone all hours of the day and night. Such a deal!

This is an area of call that is often overlooked and sometimes difficult to define contractually. Group practices in competitive areas may take call for their own patients at all times to avoid losing a patient to a colleague/competitor. And if you are a private practice physician the local group may refuse to answer your patient's phone calls or there may not be anyone nearby qualified to take the calls.

With regard to practice coverage:
1. Ask the hospital and other providers how calls are handled. If it's not clear—ask more questions. Don't assume that the other providers in your specialty are willing to cover your patients or have you cover for them.
2. Unless you want to take all your own calls, expect that having your calls covered will come at the price of covering

3. Find out if there is an answering service and how calls are screened. A good answering service might deflect emergencies to the ER, and truly nonurgent questions can be held until business hours.
4. If an answering service is available, make sure you understand how much it costs and who covers the cost.
5. Clarify who will cover your patients in the event of your absence. If you were on-call Thursday, admitted a patient from the ER, and are scheduled to leave Friday for an Australian cruise with the family, who will take over care? Don't assume the other physicians in town will step in to help. Again, for some private physicians, this can mean hiring a locums to cover your practice if you plan to be out of town.

Dr. Van Bibber: "It came as a real shock to me when I took my first job out of residency where despite joining a group of three urologists in a town with 7 urologists total, I was on call 24/7 for my own patients. Even on nights when I was out of town at a sporting event or dinner, I was constantly interrupted by phone calls. ER call weeks were only 1/7, but I never felt the relief of being truly off."

Hours Worked

"Our physician salaries rank in the 75th percentile in your specialty nationally," your recruiter proudly trumpets. Sounds pretty good—until you learn that the average physician in your soon-to-be group works 60 hours a week and spends another 10 hours at home catching up on charting. They also take call every 3rd night and typically spend at least 1 to 2 nights per week doing add-on or emergency operations.

This scenario is very common in practices where pay is based on production. Physician reimbursement has been slashed over the last few decades, and most doctors have made up for the dramatic decrease in reimbursement by simply doing a lot more. They cram 40 to 50 patients into clinic every day, fill operative schedules to the point of bursting, stay at the office until 8 pm charting every night, and then go to the home office at 11 pm after the kids are in bed for a few more hours of EMR wrestling. None of this is inherently bad. If you know how to work hard and are willing to do it in order to increase your take-home, good for you.

The problems lie in the fact that many physicians ask about pay and trust that the numbers they are quoted will come with a 40 hour workweek. Many physicians we know work as much or more than they did in residency once out in practice. Again, that is just fine if you wish to do so. But if your lifestyle is important to you, then it behooves you to make sure that you know how much you'll make if you choose to see 30 patients/day and take an hour at the end of clinic to get notes done so you can leave a clean desk behind at 5 pm.

Chapter 6: Things You MUST and MUST NOT Do.

If you've found the perfect job, have researched the practice extensively, and are ready to enter into negotiations for employment, you've arrived at our favorite part of the process. This is also the part of the process where we see most physicians' plans fly off the rails.

We have crafted this chapter of the book to address the most common problems and pitfalls that cause physicians to lose money, time, and power over their lives. Chapter 7 has some practical details for the art of negotiation, but this chapter is more about realizing what characteristics and practices will impede or facilitate your obtaining the best deal possible. Of all that we have learned helping physicians negotiate contracts, the thing that stands out most is that most physicians are good people, and as such, are prone to being taken advantage of. We have spent hundreds of hours trying to convince physicians that it is OK to make demands or that they shouldn't trust a verbal agreement. This chapter is our best effort to convince you to act in a way that will maximize your remuneration and stave off later regret.

If you want to negotiate a better contract, get more money, have a better lifestyle, stay in your job longer, help more patients, and better serve your community, start here. Here is our list of nine things you simply MUST or MUST NOT do.

1. **As a physician looking to sign an employment contract, you MUST value your education and skill set. If you don't, you can't expect anyone else will.**

Sixteen years. That's roughly what it took for us. And for you, it was probably at least eleven. Four years of undergrad, four years of med school, and a residency of three to eight years depending on specialty, fellowship, research years, etc. That is an impressive time investment.

And then there is the money. According to studentdebtrelief.us public universities charged an average of $9,970 per year for in-state tuition and $25,620 per year for out-of-state tuition for the 2017–2018 school year. Four-year private schools averaged $34,740 per year for that same time period. Four-year totals for these three different scenarios then run approximately $40,000, $100,000, and $138,000 for in-state public, out-of-state public, and private tuition, respectively.

Again, according to studentdebtrelief.us, the average cost of medical school for a single year of study at a public school for 2017 was $32,495, and for a private school, those costs rose to $52,515. Calculate out four-year costs and throw in a meager $10,000 per year for living expenses, and you have eye-popping totals of roughly $170,000 and $250,000 in costs for four years at public and private institutions, respectively.

During residency, average salaries have risen slowly and are now around $60,000 per year. But during this time, most residents with debt will continue to accumulate interest expenses. Add on a few travel loans. The costs of testing, board certification, and licensure, and the amount of money you've *spent* in getting to your first medical job is staggering.

You must also consider the opportunity cost of a medical degree. How much money were your friends who graduated from high school, tech school or college and headed straight into the workforce making every year while you were accumulating debt? How much were they placing in retirement accounts? How much debt did they eliminate? What assets did they accumulate?

Lastly, factor in the time, effort, and energy you put into those years of medical education. At the risk of sounding like the grumpy old man who walked uphill to school both ways, it was not unusual for residents in my day to work 80 to 110 hours per week. As an intern, I was on the phone with a good friend from high school who had graduated with a degree in finance and gone to work for a large brokerage firm. I was 6 weeks into my intern year on the busy cardiothoracic surgical service and had been working 110 hours a week without a single day away from the hospital since I'd started. I commented on the fact that I hadn't had a day off in 6 weeks and how it was exhausting, and he commiserated, stating that he too hadn't had a day off in 6 weeks. I was surprised but said nothing. As we continued to talk, I realized the disconnect. He had not worked any Saturday or Sunday for the last few months but had not had a "day off" during the week during that stretch. Work-hour restrictions might now limit some of those needlessly brutal stretches, but the time spent in medical school and residency remains prodigious.

You must realize that when you negotiate your contract, you are not only seeking reimbursement for the work you are about to do but for all of the work you have already done. If you fail to aggressively seek a compensation level and package commiserate with your degree and level of training you are failing to capitalize on the time, energy, and efforts of a significant portion of your life.

2. **As a physician entertaining a job offer, you MUST be a critic, not a fan. Carefully and methodically exam all aspects of a job offer and drill down on any areas that are unclear.**

We love the Miami Dolphins...

Whew, that was cathartic. We have rooted for the Dolphins since our childhood. We grew up watching David Woodley lead the Dolphins to Superbowl XVII. Then, not too much time passed, and Dan Marino led the Dolphins to Superbowl XIX. Since that time, we've held to the faint hope that Miami would return to the Superbowl. If any of you follow the NFL, you know that the Dolphins haven't returned since. But, like any sports fan, our optimism brims as the season starts.

Being a fan takes an element of irrationality. Fan is short for fanatic. People love the things they love. There is psychology research that demonstrates the connection between fans and their sports teams as similar to how others identify with nationality, ethnicity, and gender. So, when it comes to the Miami Dolphins, no matter what power rankings or position charts show us, we expect them to beat the New England Patriots. We throw analytics, experience, expert option, and rational thought to the wind. Human nature is such that when we root for something, we lose insight.

The same happens with physicians as they look for a work position. Consider this hypothetical resident: "I love that I'm going to work in my favorite city, Punxsutawney, PN! My husband and I are from there. Punxsutawney Phil and the Groundhog Day festival are amazing, and my kids will go to school where I did. Doctor Swenson is a great guy, and I'm sure he'll be a really good partner. And that recruiter, Chad, was so genuine and nice when we had dinner, I know I can trust him. Sure, the call is 1:2, the vacation time wasn't defined in the contract, there is no 401(k) match, and the OR technology is cutting edge 1987. But, I'm sure it will all work out."

Exaggerated? Maybe. But we assure you that there is truth in the preceding paragraph. We've seen physicians blinded by their fandom. Some fall in love with the place, others the first dollar amount that is dangled in front of them. Others are charmed by the partners, recruiters, and CEOs they meet. To say this can't happen to you is to deny your Homo sapiens DNA.

3. **As a physician, you MUST recognize that your skills are transferrable and transportable and that health care systems need you. As such, you MUST NOT accept subpar or poor offers. If the job offer is bad, you do yourself and your colleagues a grave disservice by taking it.**

If you're just finishing up residency, or will in the next few years, how much do you *need* that first job? The answer is different for everyone, but most residents we know are really looking forward to getting out and getting to work. Years of debt and self-sacrifice can make physicians feel liberated by the prospect of that first real payday.

Now consider how much the group you are joining needs you? They are certainly going to tell you about the need of the community and about how busy you'll be from day one. But what happens if you don't take the job?

Unfortunately, individual physicians are now often negotiating contracts with large corporate bodies. Big companies and health care systems often hold a lot of cards, and they can be intimidating opponents. When a young physician who feels like he really needs a job lands an interview with a corporation that treats physicians like any other commodity, it can be intimidating. Can't you hear a hospital suit calling out, "Hey, we need more toilet paper. Will you run to the big-box store and grab a case? Oh, and grab an oncologist or two while you're there."

The days of setting up shop in a community and fulfilling a need are fast disappearing. They are being replaced by corporate medicine. And corporations, no matter what they tell you, are rarely interested in your needs, your potential patients' needs, or the community's needs—at least not in the personal and intimate way that you are as a physician. They want "a" doctor of "blank specialty" to take a job, fill a need, generate income, and keep the system humming. And they will make you believe that if you aren't willing to swallow whatever contract they place in front of you, there is a line behind you of docs just chomping at the bit to sign and get to work.

But, here's a secret. They really need you. Every administrator at every hospital in America last year generated a grand total of $0 in revenue. Yeah, they might have shored up a few dollars by making sure everyone jumped through the correct government hoops, but they can't bill a dime. Health care systems are completely dependent on physicians and other providers to make money. And, as a physician, if the offer in front of you isn't good, you can always go elsewhere. Unfortunately, far too many of us fail to realize this simple fact, and we cower when the corporations make their demands. We cave to their weak offers. We accept pennies for the dollars of revenue we generate, and we chastise our colleagues who speak out against the poorly compensated consumption of our talents.

4. **As a physician, you MUST consider several offers. Having only one job offer limits your ability to negotiate, restricts information flow, and may force you to accept a poor offer. If, for whatever reason, you are limited in your choices, you MUST NOT communicate that to your potential employer.**

Here is a riddle for you:

When you have three of these, you have three of these.

When you have two of these, you have two of these.

When you have one of these, you have none of these.

What are these?

All too often, we meet with residents who, strapped for time and money, fail to adequately review the job market before deciding on a position. Said physician may be aware that the small town fifteen minutes from where they grew up really needs a physician of their specialty, and so they contact the hospital or group and go for a brief interview. The contract may seem "fair," and since the offered pay has one more column of digits than their current salary, they sign on the bottom line and head to work.

That might seem like a pretty good deal, but if that same physician becomes aware that a position down the road is paying twice as much or that the hospital across town pays the same but with ten more days vacation, the previously well-thought-of deal instantly becomes less appealing. As we mentioned earlier, many physicians leave their first job after just a few years. There are many reasons for this, but we know of instances where the change occurs simply because once freed from the time constraints of residency, docs adequately review their options and find that they are not being compensated as well as they might.

Consider the effect that only entertaining one offer has on the negotiation process as well. If your potential new employer wants to play hardball, what are you going to do? We know of a physician who was in just such a situation. He had worked at a hospital for several years and wanted some advice on negotiating a better contract. We reviewed his options and made a few suggestions, and off he went. Unfortunately, he was only ever really considering working in his current location, and his employer was well aware of this. Days later, we were informed that he got absolutely nothing he asked for. With no fear at all that they might lose him, the hospital simply refused to entertain any of his demands and walked away from the table.

To think of this a different way, consider shopping for a moderately or very expensive item: A new winter coat for your job in North Dakota. That first post-residency car. The custom Les-Paul guitar you've wanted since high school. Whatever it is, how would you shop for it? Jump online and buy the first one you find? Walk into the shop, point to one you want, and hand over your credit card? Unlikely. The lengthy process of shopping would likely involve hours of research, reading reviews, and hopefully, trying on several coats, test driving several cars, or playing all the guitars at the local store a few times before making the final decision.

Figure out the riddle yet? The obvious answer is choices. When you only have one, you really have none.

5. **As a physician negotiating a contract, you MUST recognize the personality traits that can be used against you. You are probably nice. They probably aren't.**

On the first day of medical school, we had a professor with a doctorate in education who walked to the front of the room, used his body to shield the chalkboard, wrote something down, and then covered what he'd written with a piece of paper that he taped in place. He then distributed a worksheet on personality types that all 101 members of my class completed. When everyone was done, he asked for a report of the numbers of each personality type and tabulated the results on the board. I don't remember the exact percentage, but the vast majority were of a personality type associated with giving/caring/soft squishy feelings. He then ripped the paper off the board to show that he'd written down the personality type and a percentage that were almost exactly spot on. He knew, before ever distributing the questionnaire, that physicians are caring people in general.

Unfortunately, the people that you are going to deal with in your negotiations know the same thing as my erstwhile professor. You are likely a nice person. You will tend to seek equity, justice, and to provide value. You will be worried about the individuals in the community and won't want to take advantage of anyone in the course of the negotiation. You'll be worried about asking for too much money or vacation, or not taking a fair share of call, of leaving the ER uncovered, or making patients travel for services. You'll want to make sure your volumes justify your pay and that your vacations don't put too much burden on your partners. You may even feel bad about asking for more reimbursement because you want to keep burgeoning health care costs down.

The companies and practices you'll be negotiating with will NOT be worried about the same things. They will pay great lip service to many of them, but in reality, they will be worried about how *little* they can reimburse you and how *much* work they can get out of you. That really nice recruiter will convince you that he or she is a friend but likely has orders to offer bare minimums and deflect your tougher questions. Those senior partners will want you to work crazy hours to make them money but will promise elusive "partnership" as a reward. The CEOs understand that when you work hard for average or lower salaries, the companies they direct look better, and their salaries increase.

You see, many folks in the business world are not nice guys. Their results on the personality test would be completely different from most physicians. They can be cold, calculating, brutal, efficient negotiators, and they will use the personality characteristics that make you a fantastic doctor against you.

6. **As a physician negotiating a contract you MUST NOT let ego prevent you from using all available information and tools.**

The old med school joke goes:

Q: What's the difference between God and a heart surgeon?

A: God doesn't think he's a heart surgeon!

As a physician, you got where you are by being smart. Most physicians we know aren't geniuses, but they certainly know how to assimilate data and use it to answer questions. So, when confronted with any new problem, they tend to do some research, read up on the problem, and attack it with the full force of their intellect.

That is often a good thing. And, is almost certainly why you are reading this book right now. There are things you don't know about contracting and negotiating, and you are going to read this book (and maybe some others), master the information, and spank that next test!

While this will often serve you well, it can also get physicians into trouble. Physicians are notorious for making poor financial decisions because they lack the financial knowledge necessary to assess risk adequately. And small personal planes are often referred to as "doctor killers" because the self-assured, and oftentimes cocky, physician pilots fail to train and put in the work needed—relying instead on their brilliance.

In contracting and negotiations, there is also a risk of physician arrogance crashing the plane. We often see physicians wade into this complicated process ill-prepared and without any assistance, assuming that their genius will get them through. Many doctors eventually do become quite good at contract issues and negotiation, but it often comes at the expense of a few wrecked fuselages! Fortunately, most contract crashes are survivable, but the wounds (financial, social, emotional) can be quite painful and slow to heal.

7. **As a physician negotiating a contract, you MUST either get experience (read everything you can, practice, be prepared to get owned by more experienced players to start) or get help.**

> "The master has failed more times than the beginner has even tried."
>
> — **Stephen McCranie**

During residency, we played Halo® to blow off steam. This was back in the day before online gaming, so a gaming night meant we all went over to someone's house, hooked up our gaming consoles and TVs, ate nachos, and played Halo.

Our first time playing Halo was against some of our friends who were gaming veterans. The results of our first foray were embarrassing. We were consistently worked over by those with more experience. That's when we learned what the word newb (short for newbie) meant. In short, we were newbs and served as video game fodder to those better than us that night. Over the next few years, we both purchased gaming systems, practiced a lot, and in the end, were competitive. But it took time, practice, and dedication to getting better.

So now, let's face it. Unless you've had experience with physician contract negotiation, you're a newb. Contract negotiating experience in the real world is hard to come by, and learning the intricacies of financial contracting isn't like learning the buttons on a gaming controller. You're certainly not going to find it nearly as enjoyable. You must understand that wisdom comes from experience, and experience comes from bad judgment. And as you negotiate what may be your first employment contract, you are likely lined up against a team of experts who has done this hundreds or thousands of times.

Remember, in the case of contract negotiation, if you suck, you don't just respawn in ten seconds. You get a hard life reset that can have a decades-long impact.

8. **As a physician, you MUST understand that because trust is an inherent part of our training, others may play this to their advantage. When you negotiate your contract, you MUST NOT be too trusting. Anything of importance MUST be in writing.**

Because of the history of the medical profession, the rigors of our education, training, and specialty certification, many people trust us implicitly. Having someone's trust is really cool. As physicians, we try every day to keep that trust sacred and be true to the Hippocratic oath. And, for the most part, we trust the majority of our physician colleagues in matters of medical decision-making.

As physicians, we also feel like comrades. We have similar shared experiences, fought the same battles, waded the same streams, braved the same minefields. And, despite our desire to practice evidence-based medicine, our training is often based on following the professional advice or opinion of an attending or some other specialist because they are one of us and are therefore deserving of our trust.

With this level of trust built into what we do professionally, it can be tempting to place trust in colleagues or administrators when negotiating a contract. However, in matters of business and money, you just can't trust others to make decisions that are best for you. Let's repeat that a bit differently: Don't trust others to make decisions that are best for you. And, if you have no experience in this type of decision-making, you might not even want to trust yourself.

You must also realize that lies and half-truths permeate every area of business—including medicine—and the promises of timeoff, autonomy, call coverage, benefits, etc., that are spoken and not written are worth the air they float on.

9. **When negotiating a contract as a physician, you MUST NOT try and decrease health care costs by accepting a lower reimbursement package.**

In the Disney/Pixar movie *The Incredibles*, Bob Parr (Mr. Incredible's alter ego) is working to aid an elderly client in distress and offers clues to navigate the complexities of the insurance industry—much to the chagrin of his boss. The subsequent lecture Bob receives includes the following line: "We're supposed to help *OUR* people. Starting with our stockholders, Bob! Who's helping them out, huh?"

Bob's boss is made out to be the bad guy in the movie: uncaring, heartless, focused only on profits. And, in our experience, physicians who talk about or focus on remuneration are similarly cast as villains. And who is the helpless little old lady in that health care scenario—the hospitals, insurers, and health care systems, of course. The CEOs and CMOs with whom you are negotiating your contract then become the Bob Parrs of the story, the heroes, valiantly trying to stave off health care cost increases and protect the poor, helpless health care system.

We have several issues with this line of thinking.

First: If you think physician reimbursement is the reason for skyrocketing health care costs, we ask you to explain the graph below. (Graph1) Hospitals and big health conglomerates are making a lot of money and funneling it to the CEOs and managers in those systems. Many so-called nonprofits really aren't; they are all about profits. Profits for the CEO, CFO, shiny new buildings, 14 vice presidents, mid-level managers, nurse managers, front-line administrators, etc. A more fitting name would be "not-for-your-profit" organizations.

Second: Physicians are THE driving force behind health care and only when providers see patients, order tests, make diagnoses, and offer treatments is money made in health care. We understand the need for capital, buildings, facilities, leadership, and all of the other cogs that make the machine of medicine work. But without providers, there is no fuel for this engine.

Third: When physicians buy into the philosophy that they must make health care affordable by accepting lower salaries and thus receiving lower remuneration than they should, they end up hurting not just themselves but their colleagues and the profession as a whole. When you take a job with Incredible Health Co. for $250,000 a year, despite data that says you should be making $350,000/year, you lose! The doc down the street loses! And in the end, the community might lose as well, as talent goes elsewhere or moves out of medicine completely because of declining reimbursement.

Health care isn't the little old lady. CEOs aren't the heroes. And doctors that demand remuneration aren't the bad guys. In the

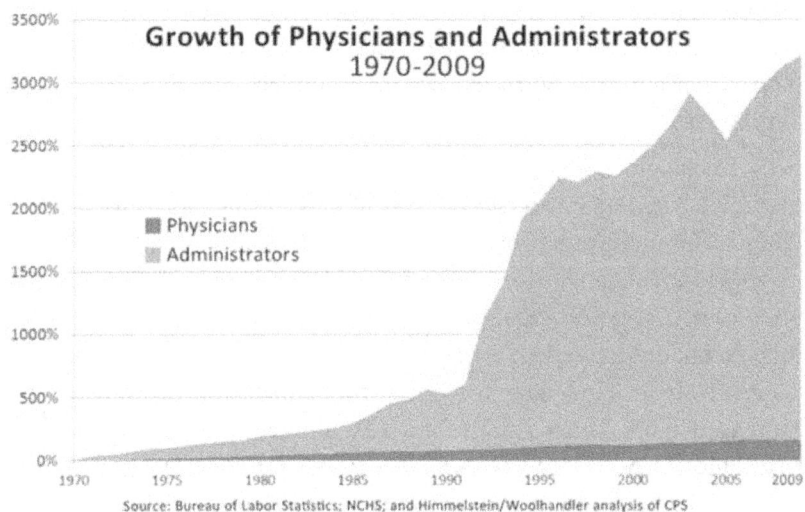

Source: Bureau of Labor Statistics; NCHS; and Himmelstein/Woolhandler analysis of CPS

end, docs who demand the pay they deserve might actually keep physicians in medicine and help stave off the coming physician and specialist shortages.

We do believe that physicians should be conscientious of health care costs. But we would argue that efforts in this area should focus on practice patterns and health care delivery optimization, not a salary reduction.

10. **As a physician, you MUST become comfortable talking about reimbursement and the business of medicine. You MUST NOT let the criticism of others prevent you from advocating for your best interests in every area.**

As a urologist, one is often referred patients who have problems that are not completely urologic in nature. A man with a rash on his back or legs or arms or head or feet or abdomen or buttocks will be sent to a dermatologist. A man with a rash on his penis is sent to a urologist! Why do you think that is? We are convinced that it is because people are uncomfortable with the penis and don't want to look at it, touch it, or think about it. Even many of our patients seem reluctant to look too closely at what is going on below the belt, and when you ask them to pay attention, look at the problem, or feel what you are feeling, they sometimes become defensive and upset. We have discussed this with our OB-GYN colleagues, and they face a similar issue.

To bring this analogy to head, let us tell you that the genitalia of medicine is remuneration. Head to your favorite medical info page and enter a comment regarding reimbursement. You'll soon have hordes of angry physicians informing you (with the caps lock engaged, of course) that you are a disgrace to the noble profession of healer and that you should consider a career in venture capitalism if that is all you care about! How dare you comment on declining reimbursement, increased work hours relative to pay, or the corporate takeover of medicine. In reality, what they are saying is that talking about the business of medicine is uncomfortable, and they don't know how to reconcile their very personal beliefs about the calling of medicine with the reality that without payment, few would or could pursue this elevated calling.

Many of the physicians we meet who stamp their feet and protest loudly at the mention of payment for services in medicine fit into two categories: the rich and the old. The wealthy, or the children of the wealthy (as is often the case), may have the luxury of taking a more meager salary due to lower debt burden, greater opportunities provided by familial money, and expectations of eventual inheritance. We know those in these circumstances who will often select their jobs based on location and schedule. The elder statesman physicians often have the advantage of having worked through decades of medicine when reimbursements, adjusted for inflation, were much higher than they are now and when patients respected their doctors. And, having secured their fortunes and enjoyed the regard of others, they are now happy to accept diminished reimbursement and call out any who refuse to do so. To be clear, we do not begrudge the privileged their dollars or the seasoned their respect. But we will argue vehemently with any who try and shame young physicians from maximizing their earnings.

It is not uncommon to see a group of physicians march into an administrator's office and demand a new piece of equipment or a certain brand of devices. But ask the same group to work together to increase reimbursement, and they will all look at their shoes or the ceiling and push away from the discomfort such topics bring. Again, don't look at that penis!

Whether we like it or not, medicine is a business. It always has been. Ol' doc Potter might have taken care of young Jimmy for a few eggs and a scrawny chicken, but a transaction occurred nonetheless. Many, if not most of us, will give our services away for free from time to time. But we should choose when that happens! And, we believe that the well-compensated physician is better able to decide when and how to provide charity care.

Chapter 7: The Art and Science of Negotiation

If you haven't done it already, and even if you have, read or reread chapter six. Many of the physicians we know are caring, compassionate, kind, considerate, thoughtful, measured, and devoted. If you were asked to describe the characteristics of a great negotiator (the policeman negotiating the release of a hostage or the business titan negotiating the sale of his business), you would likely come up with a different set of adjectives.

The good news is that you don't have to change who you are to be a better negotiator. Learning to negotiate doesn't mean you become some tough as brass hardnose, but you may need to learn a new vocabulary and change the way you would otherwise say things. At work, we feel that you should always keep your compassion focused on your patients, with ample portions given to the physicians, nurses, CNAs, MAs, etc., with whom you work. In negotiation of your contract, we would encourage you to save a little compassion for yourself, your spouse, your children, your future grandchildren, and the charitable organizations you plan to fund along the way and demand the absolute best you can get. When you see things this way, the demands you're making (with steely resolve) won't seem "mean," they'll seem appropriate.

In the early stages of creating Contract Doctors (our physician contract negotiation service), we went to Cambridge, Massachusetts, and attended the Harvard Program on Negotiation (PON) in association with the Harvard School of Law. In this three-day course, we met individuals from all areas of industry, attended lectures from top negotiators, and had opportunities to participate in workshops and negotiation practice sessions that were enlightening. We have subsequently spent hundreds of hours reading books on negotiation and reviewing our notes from the courses we attended and hundreds more hours helping physicians work through their individual contract negotiations.

Negotiation, as it turns out, is a science and art unto itself. It can be learned. There is a vocabulary associated with the effective practice of the craft, and one can prepare for and practice negotiation like any other discipline.

We realize, however, that residency is often like holding down two full-time jobs, and clinical practice can be just as busy. As such, you might not have the time to attend a three-day course or read a slew of books on negotiation. Additionally, you may simply not be interested in becoming a good negotiator. You certainly didn't go into medicine because of your love of making a good deal!

If you are interested in learning more about negotiation, we cannot recommend the Harvard Program on Negotiation course strongly enough. If you are interested in books on negotiation we would suggest you start with *Never Split the Difference: Negotiating As If Your Life Depended on It* by Chris Voss and *Getting to Yes: Negotiating Agreement Without Giving In* by Roger Fisher.

If you are not interested in negotiation as a field of study, we understand. We hope to provide for you a list of items to consider that will allow you to avoid being taken advantage of and committing the life malpractice we mention in chapter one. This list is far from exhaustive, and many of the points made here would be subjects of separate chapters in a tome dedicated solely to the art of negotiation. But, if you are a busy physician or resident who wants the nickel version, here are a few pointers.

1. Prepare to negotiate by listing and organizing the aspects of your potential job offers that are most important to you. Consider the alternatives you have to the deals you are working on.

2. Don't be afraid to negotiate the negotiation. Outline timelines, confirm individuals that will be making decisions

(CEOs vs. recruiters), and specify verbal or written communication as your preference for your discussions.

3. Ask questions that will get others to work on your problems and solve them for you. Instead of saying, "I need salary X!" ask, "How can I be expected to make this move when what you're offering is lower than salary X I'm being offered elsewhere." To help with this, try and start your questions with "what" and "how."

4. Be respectful of the parties with whom you negotiate and constantly focus on the areas of conflict, not the individuals in the process. When you have discordant demands, don't take it personally and never hold it against the person with whom you are dealing. Invite your "adversary" to work on the problem with you. Attack the issues, not the people. As an example: If you want more vacation and your potential employer is fixed on a lesser amount, try and focus on the disparity. "I'd sure love to work here, Mr. Smith, and the salary and benefits package seems fair. How can *we* come to an agreement on this vacation issue?"

5. Have a reason for your numbers, and remember that "I want it" is not a reason. Don't get hung up on the anchor (the first number offered by your negotiation counterpart), and consider offering your own number as an anchor early in the negotiation only if you have a good knowledge base.

6. Never bid against yourself. Don't move from your position until there is a counter.

7. Ask for more than you want, and be prepared to surrender items that are of little importance to you. A lot of money is left on the table of medical negotiation for lack of a simple request.

8. Make initial offers in the form of a range and shoot high. When you say: "I think an annual salary of $700,000 to $800,000 per year is a reasonable target," the opposite party will hear the high end of your proffered range and

often move in that direction. Overshoot your end goal/target with the lower number and let the higher number in your range run loose.

9. Never provide your absolute limits. If you inform your future employer, "I'd be willing to take $250,000, but I'd sure like $300,000," you should expect to settle at the lower amount.

10. When making final offers be very specific and consider using odd numbers. Requesting a salary of $437,977 may lead others to believe you've done some heavy thinking and have come up with a firm number to which they are more likely to agree.

11. Negotiate the whole package. Don't focus solely on the salary, and try and scrap together your other demands later. Make sure the ENTIRE deal is what you want before you agree to sign.

12. Don't be afraid to walk away from a deal if it's not what you want. Sometimes no deal is the best deal you can make.

13. Research your negotiating counterpart and find out if they have a history of working with and meeting demands. If negotiating with Impressive Health Corp, you'll likely have much less leverage than with a regional or community hospital.

14. Learn to recognize the following difficult negotiation tactics and avoid simply surrendering to them or quitting the negotiation because of them. Respond by listening carefully, paraphrasing, and looking for ways to change the scenario to your favor. If you see these tactics being used against you, consider taking a break before you get upset.

    A. Take-it or leave-it offers
    B. Claims of no authority (i.e., The CEO and Board will have to make that decision)
    C. Outrageous initial offers

- D. Hands-are-tied strategies (i.e., That's the way it always works here)
- E. Deadlines (i.e., We need to know by tomorrow)
- F. Emotional manipulation (i.e., Don't you care about the patients?)

15. Practice your negotiation. Get a friend or coworker and role-play the negotiation.
16. Negotiate with yourself first. You can't negotiate with others if you aren't honest with yourself about how much you're willing to give or take in the process.
17. Get qualified help. We can't emphasize this enough. Find someone that has gone through the process and that you trust to help you along the way. Remember that the attendings and individuals you would often turn to for help might have no experience in this field, and their advice may be detrimental.

Epilogue

Dr. Barton has a dog named Dash. As a puppy, whenever Dash saw himself in a mirror, he snarled and got ready for a fight. As an observer, this frequent growling and snarling was often comical but, with time, became frustrating. How could Dash repeatedly mistake his harmless reflection for a foe worthy of aggression?

As we evaluate physician contracts and watch doctors discuss remuneration, we often have the same sense of bemusement and frustration. Why do physicians seem to be constantly posturing for a fight with an opponent that outside observers might have difficulty differentiating from the original combatant? What can we learn from Dash?

First, as an individual, it can be hard to look at yourself and recognize your own shortcomings. Dash didn't recognize the dog in the mirror. And similarly, many physicians seem to be able to peer into the mirror of self-reflection and not recognize what is looking back. I'm sure we are all aware that arrogance exists in our profession. There are studies on the arrogance of physicians. If you read that last statement and had the thought, "No way! I'd like to see those studies!" then you might be in trouble. Dwelling on shortcomings isn't a productive way to effectuate change. But, we must realize that some of our shortcomings hinder our individual ability to navigate employment negotiation.

In our time working with doctors on negotiating terms of employment, we've met some wonderful people. It's safe to say that many of these people are far more intelligent than we are. However, one thing we have that our clients lack is training and experience. Yet, despite this, we've had several clients refuse our counsel. They have wanted to go at the problem their way. For whatever reason, they would retain us for services, receive consulting, then argue with our recommendations. Then, when things didn't go as envisioned, they were critical of our performance. After these experiences, we looked at ourselves, our methods, and our recommendations with a critical eye. This was insightful.

We all need to be better at looking in the mirror. See ourselves for who and what we are. Assess our strengths and weaknesses. Be realistic about what we don't know. Then, educate ourselves and improve. We should be careful not to gloss over shortcomings and become our own enemy! Let's not be like the young dog that snarls and gets ready to attack his own reflection. Having seen our reflection let's take note and calmly work on improvement.

Second, as a group, physicians seem to have difficulty working together. Physicians aren't good about agreeing on things. How many times have we sat in grand rounds and watched physicians discuss (hopefully not argue) over the proper way to handle a clinical condition? How many times have we personally defended our position in a similar setting? How often do you stand up for a patient in the ICU, on the floor, in clinic, against an insurance company, or just because no one else will? Individually, we have become good at defending our positions. It takes backbone to do what we do.

However, this strong individualism can also become an Achilles' heel when it comes to contract negotiation. We all know there is strength in numbers. Yet, the current model is for young residents with no experience to speak of to go at contract negotiations alone. So, why don't we have mechanisms through which we can unite for the common goal of making our jobs and lives better? And what are the solutions to the fractured nature of physician contracting?

One possible solution to this problem would be unionization. This topic, like so many in this book, could fill tomes on its own. There is a concise summary on the legalities of physician unionization found at medicaljustice.com

To quote: *Physicians who are hospital employees (or collective employees of a different large organization) may unionize. Physicians still in training now have an enforceable right to unionize under the National Labor Relations Act. Independent physicians who attempt to unionize will likely violate anti-trust laws.* https://medicaljustice. com/can-doctors-form-a-union/#:~:text=In%20summary%3A%20 Physicians%20who%20are,likely%20violate%20anti%2Dtrust%20 laws.

Can you imagine the power physicians would have if they banded together to negotiate? It's a thought worth considering, but as we see it, there are two main problems with physician unionization.

First, it's generally considered unethical for physicians to strike. As we considered the thought of a labor strike, the potential impact on patients was discussed, and we dismissed the possibility outright. We (like most, if not all of you) could never walk out on patients for the purpose of forcing a salary negotiation. In the event that a physician strike did occur, we can only imagine that public sentiment on Twitter and Facebook would not put the picketing doctors in a very flattering light.

Second, as physicians, we probably couldn't agree with one another enough to collectively bargain anyway. Herding cats, leading roaches, pick your metaphor. Physicians are notoriously individualistic, and our own experience would tell us that consensus on even small issues would be hard-won.

Suffice it to say that collective bargaining as physicians has traditionally been regarded as unrealistic and will likely remain so.

Considering individual and group dynamics, as mentioned previously, it becomes obvious that a big part of the problem is us! We sabotage ourselves with inadequate preparation and business education. We fight with each other based on loyalties to factions of specialty or within departments. Colleagues of the same specialties will fight overpayment based on tenure and age. We are so focused on trying to get the biggest piece of the scrap the health care companies, insurance companies, and government payers throw us we've lost sight of the meal on the table.

Unfortunately, this lack of preparation and the incessant infighting is exploited. Increasing numbers of administrators and managers sit down to the table and feast upon our work. We miss their entry and don't see their feast because we're still fighting for the scrap on the floor.

There are reasons that physicians' salaries are dropping while hospital CEOs are getting paid more. There are reasons that physician burnout is accelerating. And we believe that physician indifference and avoidance of contracting and financial matters is one of those reasons and deserves to take a significant portion of the blame. Too dramatic? Maybe. But, where would we be as a profession with unity? Go ask your dentistry buddies about their professional organizations and political activism for the specialty. You may be surprised in what you learn. It is our firmly held belief that if we don't find a way to start helping each other, there will be no one left to help.

So what can be done if unionization is out of the question and collective bargaining seems impossible? Even outside of medicine, in fields where unionization is common and possible, many workers would prefer to negotiate their own contracts and not be beholden to a union or collective agreement. We can take solace in this and realize that the ultimate power behind the contracts we sign and deals we make lies with us. We believe that the best and most reasonable possible solution is for physicians to educate themselves and strive to communicate with one another to ensure the best contracts possible, all while maintaining contractual independence. Doctors must find ways to negotiate individually with group concerns in mind. Education on business and contracting, cooperation between and among specialties, sharing of compensation information, refusing uncompensated work, and looking out for the interests of colleagues could change the way and amount all physicians are reimbursed.

As Dash grew older, he stopped growling at his own reflection and made peace with the interloper in the mirror. He learned. We sincerely hope that as individual physicians and as a collective group of healers, we can be as wise as Dash.

We hope this book will provide physicians with information to better understand their job options, to better understand themselves, and to negotiate deals that will allow them to have long, productive, and happy careers. We hope that this work will open lines of communication and get physicians to openly discussing the future of medical reimbursement as well as the future of medical care. We sincerely care about our fellow providers, and we want them—you!—to be valued for what they do. We have one of the noblest and most challenging professions in existence. Let's work together to keep it that way.

See you on the wards, and good luck going forward!

Sincerely,

Mike and Jared

www.ingramcontent.com/pod-product-compliance
Lightning Source LLC
LaVergne TN
LVHW011730060526
838200LV00051B/3110